The Truth about Migraines to Multiple Sclerosis and More

What Your Doctor Isn't Telling You But Science Has Proven

Barbara J. Tancredi BSc, CN

FRONT COVER Photograph provided by Dr. Naweed I. Syed (FRCP Edin), Professor and Head Cell Biology and Anatomy, Research Director Hotchkiss Brain Institute, Faculty of Medicine, University of Calgary.
Photo description: Growth cones of extending neurites are labeled with cytoskeletal proteins action (red) and
tubulin (green). These are healthy neurites *before mercury*. See photo of neuron being damaged by mercury in
Chapter 9 *Multiple Sclerosis*.

Cover design by Booksurge Publishing www.booksurge.com

This book can be ordered at www.amazon.com or directly from the publisher
www.booksurge.com Quantity discounts are available.

ISBN 1-4392-2514-1

~ Acknowledgements ~

My thanks

...to my momma Kathie Newman for reading the entire first draft
and making such wonderful suggestions and corrections

...to my dear friend Bill Lynam for reading the entire
second draft and nitpicking quite nicely

...to my best friend, partner in life and husband Ralph
for loving me so much more than anyone deserves to be loved and
insisting upon being the first to read this book

...to my three beautiful children Gina, Tony & Francesca
for coming into my life and making it worthwhile
and who I pray *never* suffer

...to Travis, Eric and Gina Marie for increasing my joy

...to my precious granddaughter, Giuliana,
may you always feel glorious and experience all the joy
and accomplishments for which God put you here

...to Tom & Karen, Julie & Chris, Jonathan & Kevin,
Jeanine & Dale, Jared & Jacob and Michelle & Derek for
being the most supportive, loving and generous
family on earth

...to all the doctors (and you know who you are) who hired me and
gave me such interesting things to learn and do

...and above all to God for entrusting me with truth

TABLE OF CONTENTS

Chapter 2

Chapter 3

Chapter 7

Chapter 8

Chapter 9

Chapter 10

Chapter 11

Chapter 12

INTRODUCTION

Who These Truths Are For

The truths I write about are likely not going to be understood by the 18 year old suffering from a few pimples, nor by the 20 year old with occasional menstrual cramps. Also these truths are not yet for the 24 year old young man who suffers from a bad sore throat two or three times a year but otherwise feels so good he can't remember what pain feels like in-between. Likewise, and much to my surprise, these truths aren't even for those who suffer, say with migraines, but who would rather risk staying on the path to worse things (like multiple sclerosis or stroke) because, for now, the drugs their doctor gives them take away the pain, and that's easier than sacrificing the eating or drinking of anything they wish.

No, these truths aren't anything these folks would likely comprehend right now. Perhaps they feel more good than bad, and making any changes "costs" more than the perceived benefits. However, these truths are for *all* of the above one day, likely sooner than they realize. Unfortunately, they may only "get" it when they feel a strange lump in their breast, or they start having life-changing migraines, the kind that make you want to die, and *no amount of medicine* takes the pain away. Sadly, these truths may only resonate with that young man when he gets a sore throat that doesn't go away anymore and he goes to the doctor and the bottom falls out of his world, because the doctor says he has throat cancer. Yes, these truths may be of interest to those folks then — and hopefully it won't be too late.

Of course, any day, any one of us can go to the doctor feeling "not right", and be told we have lupus, or Lou Gehrig's Disease, multiple sclerosis or cancer. The truth is, it's happening to *more* than every other person, every day (See Chapter 2 *One Out Of Two People*).

For now, these truths will likely be mostly comprehended and accepted by people that non-suffering people don't even see or know. They don't see or know them because the sufferer is either confined to their home, lying in a hospital bed, or may even be sitting next to them at work – but the *last* thing that sufferer wants anyone to know is that they have cancer, or the beginnings of Alzheimer's, or multiple sclerosis or Parkinson's. I'm writing this mostly because I want my years of education, experience, and above all, my years of suffering, to generate truths that can be etched in stone for future generations to use as a handbook of "what *not* to do". If I could spare my own children any suffering I'd lay down my life right this minute. I need to impress upon them the importance of avoiding toxic substances as the demons they are, and to not become complacent to toxins just because they are "common".

But I'm also writing this for every person who deals daily with debility, worry or pain, wondering if they'll be able to withstand the torment if it gets worse. Unfortunately, people who don't understand how bad it can get, merely think illness is a part of living out their normal lifespan. For those who haven't experienced daily suffering, they think that to suffer means to hurt, take "something" to not have pain, and then eventually die. But people who truly suffer know that you don't just get sick and then you die - that would be way too easy. Too many people suffer *unbearably* to where it is a blessing when they leave this earth. Unfortunately, before getting to that point, some of these are people who are still going to work, but wonder how long until they'll be confined to a wheelchair or a hospital bed – or of course, even dead. So who am I writing this for? If you've ever thought your pain was too great to endure, wondered how and why you got to a point of chronic suffering, and just *know* there has to be a reason or reasons that doctors aren't telling you - these truths are *definitely* for you.

I realize that for many, "death" is a nasty word. But for those who have suffered many illnesses for many years, it's never far from their mind. Thankfully, the Bible says that anyone who doesn't think about death is a fool. It also says that the day you die is better than the day you are born. I personally *cling* to those "promises". Indeed, having suffered through countless 10+ migraines, the thought of feeling *nothing* has been something for which I've prayed. Of course I'd much prefer a complete healing, but the Bible also says that God knows the exact time and day we will each die. So I take great comfort in knowing that *everyone* must die. I take even greater comfort in knowing that God is in control, and part of that control is when we play by God's rules we benefit. Above all, I have figured out that God's rules are being profoundly broken by modern civilization as we consume foods full of glutamates, inject ourselves with mercury and satisfy thirst with alcohol or soda.

I've prayed many times during my greatest pain that my pain *not* be for nothing. I've prayed that what I've been through and what I've learned may help others know what to do and not do. What I've learned above all, physically, is that pollutants are *causing* our diseases, that parasites are opportunistic and *contributing* to our diseases. All the diet, supplements and therapies in the world won't work to heal you to any degree if the pollutants and parasites are not *eliminated*.

Radical Measures For Radical Healing

radical adj. Arising from or **going to a root or source**; basic: proposed a **radical** solution to the problem.

Here's an illustration regarding what "radical" means. Even though after 911, President Bush exclaimed, "America is addicted to oil", then a couple of years later made a similar cry – it doesn't appear anyone has done anything to even come close to *beginning* to solve the problem. A July, 2008 CNN special "Out of Gas" says the "clock is ticking" and we're a lot more vulnerable than we want to admit. Sudden $4.50-$5.00/gallon gas prices has proven this. The show goes on to talk about how quickly these price spikes came upon us, and we're simply not prepared to operate any way but by our (America's) current consumption of a quarter of the world's entire production of oil/gas. The film plays "devil's advocate" and makes "news announcements" as if it were really happening right now. The news announcements are of trucks not being able to get to the stores; of over a fourth of all stores empty and closed; of the airline and touring industries all bankrupt, etc.

Richard Branson of Virgin Airlines has businesses that all run on oil. A few years ago he was motivated to want his own refinery. Al Gore and others jumped on him right away and told him that's not the way to a permanent fix of the problem. They convinced him that growing corn to make ethanol would be the way of the future. So Richard Branson put billions into growing corn and creating ethanol. This has backfired miserably. It turns out that growing the corn uses as much energy as it produces!

The documentary goes on to say, "But there is one country that made a hard decision several decades ago, and has *solved* its energy problem". I have to tell you I was on pins and needles until the commercials ended so I could hear <u>what</u> country, and <u>what</u> they have done. Well, it's Brazil, and three decades ago they started growing sugar cane to produce ethanol. Apparently it's far more energy-efficient to grow than corn. But more importantly *all* their cars are now "flex" cars and can run on ethanol. Currently (2008) Brazil doesn't import *any* oil/gas.

So how does this story relate to healing? It relates because radical measures for radical healing means *getting to the core or the true cause of the problem* – no matter what the cost. For lawmakers, pharmaceutical manufacturers, doctors, etc., it could very well mean forgoing profit in favor of giving people the whole truth and nothing but the truth about what is causing their illness (and therefore, what they need to do to prevent and cure illnesses).

For example, if all a doctor needs to do is tell you about an herb that heals your condition, they could lose millions, even billions in drug sales if everyone stopped buying the drug. How can *you* turn this profit-based system of "health care" around? Well, to get to a point of knowing the true cause of your problems would require tireless effort on your part. It may mean refusing to buy anything that *doesn't* address your core issue. This may mean refusing a doctor's prescription until he can tell you exactly what's wrong with you, and exactly *how* what he is prescribing works, while simultaneously guaranteeing that his prescription has zero risk of harming you! Can this happen? Not until everyone rises up and demands it, because the truth is, what is driving our "health care" industry is the most profitable thing, not the safest and best thing. Hard to believe, but I've been at the core of it for years and have heard the doctors talking about so-and-so's insurance and ability to pay – *not* how can we cure their condition.

But you prove this every time you buy the cheaper item made in China over the more expensive item made in U.S.A., especially after you've been hearing of product after product from China tainted with lead or other deadly toxin! The truth is obscured because money is nearly always the bottom line instead of the absolute truth. If not, we'd have millions of solar cars on the road already. Solar cars are currently being used in races across Australia, and in experimental golf carts. There have been models of solar cars, but few yet produced for consumer purchase. It's not "free" energy, because they are costly to produce, but it's renewable energy, and protective of the environment to boot.

Unfortunately, often for those that know the truth, that is, they know what would best help them heal, affordability is a limiting factor. For example, you may know that stem cells will help you, and that they are available in another country, but the trip, time away from work, and price of the stem cells are prohibitive.

I know people who will say its more complicated than all of the above. But I also know about doctors not getting to the bottom of health issues because all they'd have to do is tell you to "just go home and heal". So why don't they? They *don't* do that because they know they'd collectively lose billions if everybody just "went home to heal". So contrarily, I know firsthand that solving many of our problems is likely *less* complicated than anyone would have you think. Instead of solar or hydro energy, or harnassing the wind, GM is now producing an entirely electric car, which of course requires that we build more electric plants, most of which will end up being nuclear. *More targets for terrorists?* Not only that, there are engineering issues, like the tendency for an electric car to have a "thermal event" (a fire). Of course this is all why we need to humble ourselves and look to God. What energy has God given us freely and abundantly? Three that come to mind immediately are wind, sun, and running water. Speaking of which, in the news, 2008, there are several stories appearing about the "compressed air" vehicle!

Of course there is also our own leg power. We need major incentives for people to both work at home and to work close to home so they can walk or bicycle to work! The health and environmental benefits would be *enormous!* We also need to harnass the aforementioned solar, wind and water power. This is all to say, that *it takes radical measures to obtain radical results.*

With regard to your health, you may find it to be a "radical" step to re-do half of your dental work (see Chapter 6 *Dental Work*) because it may be causing or contributing to your diseases and pain. Yet that may be exactly what you need! And why doesn't your dentist or doctor tell you this? Your doctor just might lose a patient. And your dentist makes thousands per *tooth* when you undergo their disease-contributing procedures like root canals and crowns. For me, amalgams began my spiral into the depths of health hell on earth *and* the removal of all dental toxicities has been one of the very *best* things I've ever done health-wise (more about this later).

I intend to continue the journey of healing, but only by looking to the truth, the whole truth, and nothing but the truth. And God (the author of Nature) is the author of all truth. I'd love for you to go on this journey with me – the more the healthier. In fact, if you want this truth to help as many people as possible, send me your story of healing by getting to the root cause. You have to know that if millions of people band together with similar stories, we would threaten the "big business" of medicine and pharmaceuticals. Be prepared for that – people that make *big* money aren't at all happy when it is threatened. Indeed, health-care professionals have everything to lose if 80-90% of diseases simply disappear because the mercury and other poisons that are causing them are no longer being used.

Note: As you read through this book, you'll note that there are scientific studies as well as quotes of other authors within "text boxes" throughout. The purpose of the text box is to separate the more complicated material from the rest of the text. If you are like me, and find people or studies that back up, hypothesize or even prove what is being said, you will find the text boxes helpful, even exciting. For those who don't care about authorities or "science", you can mostly choose to skip over the text boxes.

This is an "interactive" book. There are many references pointing you to books, videos, websites and more giving you tangible information that will shed light on truths people simply aren't being told. These reference aids will help you in your quest for healing, as well as in educating supportive family and friends. Consider each link, book or video critical for a more complete understanding.

My intention is to provide the reader with scientific truths along with common sense, as well as personal experience. From these truths, each reader needs to make his/her own decisions and choices. In addition each reader needs to continue his/her own research. If any reader decides to try the diet, supplements or other suggestions in this book, it is entirely their own choice. Of *course* I thoroughly believe in (and indeed, have proven) every word I've put forth. I have also experienced the efficacy of the diet, supplements and avoidance of factors that cause disease. That said, I can in no way be responsible for anyone else. Proceed with a bit of intelligence, a lot of wisdom and complete responsibility for yourself. Let the truth, and only the truth, guide you and give you courage.

DEDICATION TO MY CHILDREN

And To *Your* Children

    Please don't pollute your body. For example, cadmium (a toxic heavy metal) in cigarettes will ultimately destroy your body's ability to effectively fight parasites (e.g., bacteria, fungi and viruses) which will cause far worse things than cold sores and sore throats! Alcohol is very damaging to your body's cells, literally killing liver cells, and shriveling brain cells.

> "Cadmium has no constructive purpose in the human body. It, and its compounds, are extremely toxic even in low concentrations, and will bioaccumulate in organisms and ecosystems." *Wikipedia.*

Now add to this the daily use of radiation sources (like cell phones and computers) and it's not a matter of if - but *when* you will get throat, lung or brain cancer. Take this very, very seriously - and trust me, you don't want <u>any</u> type of cancer. You think cold sores or pimples are "annoying"!? Cancer is devastating, frightening, and far more painful than cold sores and sore throats. The quote below states within the full article that one reason you hear so many denials as to the link between cell phone use and cancer is that "heavy use" is defined as using the phone *once per week*! Who uses their cell phone only once per week?

> ...... a 2008 study by Swedish cancer specialist Lennart Hardell found that frequent cell phone users are twice as likely to develop a benign tumor on the auditory nerves of the ear most used with the handset, compared to the other ear. A separate study in Israel determined that heavy cell phone users had a 50 percent increased likelihood in developing a salivary gland tumor. In addition, a paper published this month by the Royal Society in London found that adolescents who start using cell phones before the age of 20 were **five times more likely to develop brain cancer at the age of 29** than those who didn't use a cell phone. [Scientists warn US Congress of cancer risk for cell phone use. September 2008. www.physorg.com]

Imagine going to the doctor for a sore throat that doesn't go away. Perhaps after weeks of suffering you go to the doctor and he tells you that you have throat cancer. He tells you surgeons will have to cut out parts of your throat to save your life. While he likely won't elaborate, the liklihood is that talking and swallowing may be compromised or taken away completely. You will likely look mutilated. You may have to have a tube down your esophagus so "nutrition" can be put down to your stomach to keep you alive. All because you chose to play Russian roulette with your health by smoking or using a cell phone to your head? *This happens to someone, somewhere every single day — in fact about 110 people per day are diagnosed!*

Head and neck cancer has an annual incidence of about 40,000 per year. That makes up for about 5% of the incidence of new cancers. Two-thirds of patients will present with locally or regionally advanced disease. So that's the most common presentation for throat cancer, mouth cancer, head and neck cancer, oral cancer, and tongue cancer. Traditional therapy...has been surgery and/or radiotherapy. [http://www.ccspublishing.com/journals_6a/throat_cancer.htm]

You have your entire life ahead of you! So much opportunity! With cancer, your life will likely be ended in a most horrific way. But it doesn't have to be that way. You have far more control than know!

WASHINGTON, August 4, 2000 — A Maryland neurologist has filed an $800 million lawsuit against Motorola, Bell Atlantic and others, charging that years of using a cellular phone has given him brain cancer. Chris Newman, 41, cited a 1994 study on rats that showed breaks in DNA, a possible sign of future cancer, after the animals were exposed to radiation. [http://www.consumeraffairs.com/news/doctor_sues.html]

Then, in May, 2008, another neurologist announced that cell phones *do* cause brain cancer and he issued a warning for everyone to stop using them. Keep them away from your body, he recommends. Only use text or speakerphone. In addition, do not use "Blue Tooth" or regular earphones as they also bring radiation to your head unless they are the "air tube" type (not the type you buy at the cell phone vendor — see the right kind at: www.mercola.com).

But you can bet the multi-billion dollar cell phone industry will do everything in its power to keep this neurologist from saying much more. As it was, this piece on the evening news was less than one minute long! With such alarming news, you'd think we would hear it over and over. We did not.

Years ago I saw a video of a demonstration that was done by scientists where they measured the radiation from a cell phone going through a head. It was a "dummy" head filled with a similar weight and viscosity of fluid as your brain, but they proved that the radiation goes right through to the center of the brain. This video has "disappeared". But as for me, I won't wait until the "jury" decides whether cell phones are dangerous. Risking a brain tumor isn't an option. So in keeping with using Nature as my guide (and the fact that a cell phone near my head actually hurts, and has done so long before I knew anything about the danger) I choose to keep them away from my head, and body. I do use a cell phone, but only to text (and I set it down to send the text), or with an external speaker. You can go to http://reviews.cnet.com/cell-phone-radiation-levels/ and find a chart of cell phones with the highest levels of radiation vs. those with the lowest as well.

One area young people are completely foolish about, is somehow thinking that "oh well, if I die, I die". They need to know that that's not how it works. You won't just smoke, drink, eat foods laden with chemicals and then die. You will *suffer* for years and years first — but why would you allow this? Why, indeed, when God has given you so many abilities and gifts to experience joy in this life. Deliberately allowing toxins to *destroy* it all, one cigarette (cadmium and other toxins), one drink (damages your defense systems, especially your liver), one "Top Ramen" (loaded with free glutamates that damage your central nervous system and brain) at a time is simply foolishness.

In addition, many young people believe there is no way *they* can become addicted. I'll share the story of a beautiful 40 year old gal who rented a room in my home and it quickly became obvious she was totally addicted to both cigarettes and alcohol. Her diet was made up of candy and Top Ramen according to what was in her room. She was tormented because she'd lost her husband and her two babies. She *looked* perfectly normal, and that's the devilish deceit! Sadly, within three weeks she was dead. There was not a day went by that she wasn't in the most horrific emotional pain, and judging by the pain pills in her room, in physical pain as well. She must have sensed she couldn't hold on much longer – she went home to ask forgiveness of her mother, and died that night in her mother's bed. The moral of the story? This beautiful gal didn't think she was becoming addicted when she began smoking or drinking, probably as a teenager – and that's the real tragedy. She wasn't a bad person – the substances overpowered her. Addiction sneaks up on you - like the devil.

It is my *desperate* desire to prevent you from suffering even 1/100th as much as that gal or as I have. Instead of being addicted to "substances", be addicted to all the abilities and blessings God has given you. Yet I've seen teens agonizing over a cold sore or a pimple and not want to go to work. They hurt, fret, and hate how they look and feel. I ask myself, can't you realize that the one little blemish is *nothing* compared to how you'll suffer if you keep filling your body with pollutants? Pollutants like cadmium as well as other pollutants from cigarette smoke (your own and your friends' secondhand smoke); as well as alcohol and glutamates in the foods you choose to eat daily can only lead to one thing - suffering. And don't think that you are somehow protected from harm by your ignorance.

The typical young person in America, if not the world, is doing absolutely *nothing* to give his or her body the necessary tools to fight pollutants. While there are *thousands* of antioxidants, trace minerals, quality proteins, fiber, and more, they are only available in pure, whole, fresh (preferably organic) fruits and vegetables, eaten mostly raw (cooking destroys most nutrients nearly completely). If you're looking at older folks who have been smoking for years and you think "they're fine" - think again. They are either only a "day away" from being told they have cancer (usually terminal if they've smoked their entire life), or they've eaten very well over the years (many "older folks" grew up on farms!) and all those antioxidants got them this far without succumbing yet to cancer. "Older folks" also did not grow up around all the radiation sources we have today from cell phones to microwaves. Today's generation is not so fortunate. From a diet devoid of protective nutrients, to daily bombardment with toxic radiation, heavy metals and more, young folks today can expect to succumb to horrible diseases earlier than ever. I know of a boy who has Parkinson's, and has had it since 10 years old. In addition, there are entire wings of hospitals dedicated to childhood cancers – to name just two horrific diseases.

If you continue ignoring the truth, your world will come crashing in on you much sooner than you can even imagine. And when it does, it will be too late. The damage will have been done. Once you damage your immune and neural system with heavy metals (like mercury), and your neural system with excitotoxins (free glutamates and aspartates) there may never be complete recovery. You may suffer from migraines, hearing loss, vision loss, and herpes outbreaks which causes horrific pain in your joints, hips, head, internal organs as well as contributing to neurological diseases and cancer. People are getting diseases from Parkinson's to heart disease, even having heart attacks, in their 20's and 30's these days.

One family member said to me, "It's like there's nothing that is safe anymore – we try so hard, and then in the end we die anyway!" This illustrates so well the point being missed by people who carelessly smoke and drink and "do drugs". I'll explain, using myself as the example. When toxins caused me to get psoriasis, I had a very difficult childhood emotionally, but otherwise tried to manage the best I could. Being 80% covered with ugly scales is a miserable way to grow up. But being "naturally-minded" since childhood, I turned to sweating, exercise, sunshine, and a better diet along with supplements to help me cope, and it worked. I hated the psoriasis, but I didn't hate psoriasis as much as I loved icecream, if you know what I mean. Then, when I was in my late 20's and damage from toxins caused me to start having migraines, with pain the worst I'd ever felt, and I'd have them almost weekly, lasting up to 3 days along with nausea and vomiting - just thinking, "oh well, if I die, I die" wasn't an option anymore. I had to find out what was causing them because life was hell *with* them. That kind of pain and disruption to life (I missed out on many parties, weddings, jobs...) was unbearable. *I would have rather died than suffered another migraine.* But I couldn't just throw my hands up and say, "gee, nothing is safe anymore – oh, well, I give up trying." Now, it's multiple sclerosis, and if I don't avoid the toxins, eat the right foods, and use the right supplements, the suffering is *unbearable.* So it's not about avoiding dying – not really. *It's about not suffering unbearably while you're living.*

Suffering to the point of wanting to die is not the plan God has for your life. There will be plenty of life's lessons along the way without you deliberately creating more sorrow by way of polluting your body. I promise you God has so much joy planned for you in the things you love to do, the people you love and who love you, having children and more. You must take care of your body – for the sake of all the people that love you if not simply for your own sake.

Chapter 1
40+ YEARS SEARCHING
FOR THE TRUTH

"The truth isn't always the easiest, but anything less does enormous disservice to yourself and all with whom you have relationships."

About the Author

I have spent more than half a *lifetime* battling pain and disease. Since the age of 11 my life has been more about combatting disease symptoms, pain and debilitation than almost anything else (except God and family). I have spent over $90,000 dollars (in only six years) out of pocket on medical doctors, expensive tests, chiropractors, acupunturists, nutritionists, health spas and more in search of answers. Along the way I obtained my Bachelor of Science and my certification as a Nutritionist - *looking for answers*. I didn't find my answers in any one person or place, but from "clues" I obtained in *many* places, from many people, from trial and error, and a lifetime of researching the studies: "scientific", "clinical" and anecdotal. Perhaps the most important information I gathered, however were "God clues". That's when little "miracles of fate" occur right before your eyes, that you know are from a source higher than yourself. Those have happened more times than I can relate.

All of my research became hundreds of times more fruitful after the internet became available. Just as an interesting "aside", the internet began in thought process in the 1950's. In 1969 *Defense Advanced Research Projects Agency* (DARPA) built the first network, called CARPANET. By 1981 there were over 200 organizations linked. In 1983 the military segment moved to MILNET and the non-military portion was moved to National Science Foundation's NSFNET. In the early 1990's legislation encouraged expanded commercialization of NSFNET, which became renamed as *National Research and Educational Network* (NREN). It was in this legislation that both Ted Kennedy and Al Gore played crucial roles with their votes to authorize the Government to fund the research (which vaguely explains Al Gore's statement that he "invented" the internet).

But it wasn't until Microsoft came out with "Windows" in 1995-1998 that you and I had complete and easy access to "internet", email, etc. I remember a doctor I worked for in about 1993 or 1994 all excited about "email". He was one of the *first* I knew who had it. Every day as he was "playing" on his computer sending emails to his publisher, and they responding, I thought, "this will never catch on – it's so impersonal!" I vowed I would never use "email". (Boy was I wrong!) This is all around the time that you suddenly started seeing www "dot" everywhere you went. It was on buildings and billboards and at the bottom of your TV screen. It was also on lawyers and other professionals' business cards, and I remember thinking, "what in the heck is www "dot"". Well, we've come a long, long, way to where now even an 87 year old grandpa knows what www "dot" means! I relate this just to let you know I was there – with my little "Mac" with its 500 megabyte hard drive that cost me nearly $5,000 – searching and researching all these years to weed out the garbage and gather up gems of truth.

In fact, I believe this to be one of the most important health books you'll ever read. This book has been started, and written, and rewritten for the past dozen years. I would think I had the answer, then found it wasn't true. Back to the drawing board. I wrote and I wrote, but it never made complete sense. All the puzzle pieces never quite came together into one clear picture – until an incident long ago in my life (see chapter 7 *Psoriasis*) matched up with a recent incident (see chapter 9 *Multiple Sclerosis*) and then the picture became crystal clear.

Indeed! How do I *know* what I know? How did the Wright Brothers know what *they* knew? Those two men are responsible for proving to mankind that we could fly. Did they have a Harvard degree in flying? How did man figure out he could build a fire and cook food? Did the first person whoever built a fire have a degree in "fire"? Man since the beginning of time, motivated by *intense passion* to figure something out, worked however hard, and however long it took until he *got it right*. I'm no different. I've spent the past 44 years searching and trying and studying and struggling and jumping through hoops *looking for the answers*. It all began like the Wright Brothers (or the caveman) with an *intense passion* to figure something out. Having the disfigurement of psoriasis, the horrific pain of migraines, and the debilitating and painful symptoms of multiple sclerosis to name just a few of my own maladies, has given me that passion.

The "4-point" message that this entire book is trying to convey is:

1. **Mercury is the underlying cause of migraines, multiple sclerosis, and so much more** as you will see as you read on. In fact, mercury is likely the underlying cause of many or all neurological and immunological diseases. Other pollutants like aluminum, lead, cadmium or nickel have actually been shown in studies (and caputured on video) to *not* harm neurons as mercury so readily does (see: How Mercury Causes Brain Neuron Degeneration Chapter 9 *Multiple Sclerosis*). Not that these other metals aren't toxic, however! But mercury, by virtue of being so abundant in many human uses, such as being so stupidly plastered and injected into our bodies "wins" hands down as the world's biggest health threat. Also, mercury was my own "variable". Now if you've never heard the term "variable" before, it means when everything is the same, day after day, suddenly a "variable" is introduced into your life, and *things changed*. You can immediately and easily see what caused the change. That's me — everything the same, day after day. So when I introduced something different, I knew immediately if it changed anything. As a side note, this is why I don't believe in supplements that contain multiple ingredients — if the supplement causes a

negative reaction, you won't know which of its ingredients caused it. So I take my supplements individually.

2. **Parasites** **are opportunistic and attack cells mostly after they have been damaged by pollutants.** You might say that parasites carry on the work that pollutants start. Parasites are known to feed on diseased and damaged cells, not on healthy cells. Couple that with an immune system that can no longer defend the body because of being damaged by mercury and you've got a recipe for cancer and many other degenerative diseases.

3. **Deficiencies** **leave your cells defenseless and will determine how quickly and how deeply you will succumb to disease.** Nature has put into pure, whole, fresh, (preferably organic) plant foods all the nutrients your body needs for optimum protection from neurological diseases, skin diseases, cancer and more. In fact, you *may* be surprised to learn that there are *thousands* of cell-protecting nutrients in raw plant foods, and only with sufficient consumption of these foods can you get what you need.

4. **Drugs, radiation and surgery** **never work to heal.** To truly heal you must stop what is damaging your cells, while activating internal mechanisms that stop and reverse the disease process. If you believe a drug, radiation or surgery method "healed" you, yet a few years later the same disease returns, you were never healed, but merely received respite from the disease until the factors that caused it in the first place could regroup and resurface. Contrarily, your own body has powerful healing mechanisms within (like stem cells and healing nutrients). When these healing mechanisms are tapped into, diseases can be stopped and/or reversed. Continuing to tap into your own healing mechanisms can keep the disease from returning. I was diagnosed with lymphoma in my twenties. I went on all raw foods and other natural therapies, and watched the huge lymph glands slowly return to normal size over the course of about 12 years. I've never had a reoccurance.

Recommended Reading

While this entire book refers to, often quotes from and is in accord with the books listed below, reading these books along with this book will arm you with even more truths to help you make educated choices. You also need to know that if you decide to follow the truth, you will encounter many friends and family who will think you're crazy. I warn you, you'll be on your own in your healing quest – your insurance doesn't pay for any of it. Indeed, after you've been to the doctor half a dozen times in one year attempting to merely get a name for what you have, you may even be *denied* insurance.

For years I went to doctors but never got any answers. I suppose there are people who believe they got answers or help. This book probably isn't for them. As for me, after getting nowhere with doctors, I found that by doing research of the scientific literature and comparing it to clinical, anecdotal, and my own findings, I could discern Nature's truths, uncover the cause of my illnesses and then apply detox, dietary, supplemental and therapies (natural and medical) that have halted progression and even healed my pain. I am fully aware that many people will run the full gamut of medical testing and medications, even surgery – and may only "resort" to the true way to healing after it all fails. Unfortunately, it is usually too late by then. Recommended reading:

1. **It's All In Your Head: The Link Between Mercury Amalgams and Illness.** Dr. Hal A. Huggins.
2. **The Roots of Disease: Connecting Dentistry and Medicine.** Robert Kulacz, DDS and Thomas E. Levy MD, JD.
3. **Tooth Truth.** Frank Jerome DDS.
4. **Root Canal Coverup.** George Meinig DDS.
5. **Flood Your Body With Oxygen: Therapy for Our Polluted World.** Ed McCabe
6. **Excitotoxins, The Taste That Kills.** Russel Blaylock MD
7. **Charcoal Remedies.com: The Complete Handbook Of Medicinal Charcoal and Its Applications.** John Dinsley
8. **The Poison in Your Teeth** Tom McGuire DDS
9. **Remove the Thorn and God Will Heal** Bud Curtis

Looking For The Truth

There are older people alive today who have enjoyed health so bountiful they boast they never even get headaches. For these people, their first real health problem may not have surfaced until they were well past 60, 70 or even 80. But then there are the people I'm writing about – people with bodies and brains damaged by mercury. These folks have been to the doctor, explained all of their symptoms, and their doctor authorized a "battery of tests". Sound familiar? They obediently did all the tests, and some time later returned for the "results", and were told everything was "within normal range" Then, with their symptoms still very much interrupting their life and happiness, they plead "what is it, doctor, what is *causing* my pain?" Perhaps their symptoms are horrific headaches, numbness, cramping, inability to sleep, depression, etc., but the doctor "can't find anything wrong". This person may have the beginnings of a disease that is difficult to diagnose, like multiple sclerosis, but the doctor can't find it on his "radar" yet. So years of suffering may occur before a diagnosis – and now the disease has progressed so badly that powerful and dangerous drugs are used to combat the symptoms. This happens every day to many people. I know this because I've been working with people in the medical field for over 30 years in some capacity or other. I hear the stories and the anguish, but I have also experienced it all myself.

Some of these people say that when the doctor couldn't find anything wrong with them he opened a drawer and pulled out a sample medication and as if giving them a present, gave it to them *free*, saying, "Try this". Perhaps trusting their doctor they went home and tried the medication and it either had no effect, or horrific side-effects. Then on the news (2008) was a story about doctors admitting to giving patients who complained of chronic pain – *placebo pills*. Fake pills! That's because the doctor is at a loss, because he is not looking for the right thing – most often the underlying pollutant. He knows a drug isn't going to help either, so he resorts to fake pills. God help us.

I've been the person hired to answer the phone at the doctor's office, inundated with calls of people begging for help, they would cry "that medicine didn't work" or "I'm worse" or "now I've got a new problem". I've had *doctors* tell me, "That's why they call it the "art" or "practice" of medicine." What they rarely admit to is that *you* are the guinea pig.

Indeed, young medical students enter medical school to thoroughly learn body parts, the mechanics of these parts, and the medications, therapies and surgeries approved to treat these parts – and then of course to pass the medical licensing exam. I dare say, *most* doctors spend their entire career applying what they learned in medical school, and little more, meaning, they don't spend their spare time delving into the latest research looking for the *cause* of diseases. In fact, doctors simply do not know what causes thousands of ailments. They merely know how to write out a "hopeful" drug antidote for the symptoms. Want to prove it to yourself? Ask your doctor, "what *caused* my _____". Every single time I've asked this, I was told, "*We don't know*".

That doctors don't know what *causes* diseases became most apparent to me when, while in my 20's, a doctor I had gone to, left the room after examining me, but didn't know I had tagged close behind him on my way to visit the ladies room. As I passed by him, I saw him hurriedly thumbing through his "Physicians Desk Reference" to look up what drug he could recommend to me. I assume he's been doing that all along and likely is to this day as well. I went to him to find out the *cause* of my ailment, but the truth is, he didn't have a clue, because what is causing our epidemic of diseases is neither taught in medical school, nor can be found in that Physician's Desk Reference.

My deepest respect and regard goes out to doctors (and I know a few) who are actively involved in researching the underlying cause of disease before applying any treatments. My sincere thanks also goes to doctors who, in spite of the constant threat of ridicule and scrutiny (e.g., from the FDA) use safe, natural healing mechanisms such as stem cells and nutriceuticals. Don't get me wrong. I have the greatest appreciation for *all* doctors who work tirelessly to perfect their skills at saving the lives of people who have been injured or who foolishly live their lives in such a way as to cause themselves harm (such as those who smoke). And perhaps my greatest admiration goes out to that handful of doctors and scientists who are actively fighting to abolish deadly factors involved in disease, like mercury and glutamates. I admire them most because I know that if we were truly able to abolish these factors, the *need* for doctors would plummet, and they know it.

Is The Truth In That Other "Health Book"?

There are thousands upon thousands of "health" books. About 40 years ago I began to collect as many as I could. Then, about 20 years ago a realization hit me like a lightening bolt. I realized it after meeting a prolific author of health books. He was a naturopathic doctor (ND) and professor at a university that teaches other naturopathic doctors. I was working at the time as a nutrition lecturer. I was also helping an "alternative" doctor write his books. The ND began asking me questions when he found out I had psoriasis. After his many queries I asked him, "where do you get the information for your books?" He said, "I'm an eclectic writer…I gather information from all over, for example, from people like you." This burst a huge bubble I'd had, where I ignorantly thought that he, and other authors like him, spent their time researching in a lab or medical library. It occurred to me then that the information most health books contained was already "out there". I began looking in the indexes of all my books. I decided that if I looked up any disease (especially my own: psoraisis and migraines at the time) and the book said, "**of unknown etiology**" (i.e., we don't know what causes psoriasis or migraines) then *how on earth can they advise me as to what to <u>do</u> or <u>take</u> to help alleviate, much less heal, my disease?* Indeed, what I found is that basically all of my books had "nothing new" for me.

Then, shortly thereafter, I came across a statement in another health book wherein the doctor's advice for migraines was so aggravating that I gave all but about a dozen of my books away. He said that migraines: "won't kill you, you'll get over it, just go into a quiet dark room and let it pass."

Anyone who has migraines and truly wants to know what causes them, how to prevent them or at least alleviate the suffering once you have one would likely be as angry about that doctor's take on them as I was (he's obviously *never* had a migraine). So the few health books I've kept contain at least one single profound truth and/or are either "encyclopedic" in nature, or based upon copious amounts of research — not merely the opinions of one person, even if that person is a doctor of some kind. The bulk of the ones I have are listed in the "Recommended Reading" section earlier in this chapter.

You've Got To Remove the Thorn So God Can Heal

This next section I write, in part, to show that I didn't just "fall off the turnip truck". In fact, over the past 40 years or so, I've written 4 books with an alternative doctor as well as many health newsletters and brochures. I've done extensive literary research on therapies, nutrients and diseases for doctors. I've lectured to thousands of people as a nutritionist and I was the nutrition chef for many years for a large holistic live-in clinic. I planned and cooked three healthy meals each day for the people going through the program.

But I have also been to many "health clinics" as the patient and gone through their programs including extensive hyperbaric oxygen treatments, intravenous medicines and nutrients. I had my own bone marrow stem cells transplanted as well as had $12,000 worth of umbilical cord stem cells in another country intravenously administered to me. In addition, I've taken dozens upon dozens of different herbs, supplements and amino acids after researching their potential benefit. I own or have owned nearly every manner of ozone, infrared, magnetic, massage and electrical device supposed to help heal you.

Now, you are likely beginning to think I'm boasting that I've "learned it all". Quite the contrary. What I'm saying (as you'll see in the rest of this book) is that I've learned by a *process of elimination*, mostly "what not to do". Not that the things I've mentioned aren't of any benefit, also quite the contrary. What I'm saying is, if the actual *cause* of a disease isn't removed *first*, all of the above *cannot* heal you.

This brings to mind a book I was introduced to over 30 years ago by Bud Curtis called "Remove The Thorn and God Will Heal". Bud's book is on your "required reading" list in the "Recommended Reading" section previous. I have in no way appreciated how very important it is to remove the "thorn" as I do now. This is, in part, for the same reason many people don't appreciate it – and that is, because they don't hurt enough. The effort to remove the thorn may be greater than leaving it in and suffering a while longer. But secondly, most people aren't even remotely aware of what is meant by "thorn".

Of course you can't remove thorns if you don't know what or where they are! I can attest to over 40 years of going to doctors asking them, "what *thorns* do I have? I want to remove them", but not getting any answers at all. By "thorn", of course, I was really asking what was *causing* the disease or symptoms I was having. Do you know that in 40 years, not one doctor ever had a clue as to the *cause* of any of my symptoms, diseases or pain. Indeed, did I say not one could tell me the *cause* of my disease? Many couldn't even tell me what disease I had! Usually I went home and researched like crazy and discerned what I had myself. Then, almost without fail my "diagnosis" would be verified after I'd go back to the doctor, tell him what I had, and he/she would do a test or two, and confirm my own diagnosis. Like most who are suffering I've been a guinea pig and have often suffered dire consequences from trying what doctors suggested (again, often without even knowing what I had, much less the *cause* of what I had).

So with my own disease and pain as my motivator I've never given up. I came to know that all of my trials have had a purpose. The truth is, even supplements or therapies I tried that didn't seem to benefit me at all, if I hadn't tried them I'd always wonder if there was still "*something* out there" I hadn't yet tried that would miraculously (or easily) cure me. Trust me, there are many doctors, even "alternative" or "holistic" that are *banking* on you still believing there is "something out there" so that you'll try *their* something. One alternative doctor argued with me once that he was certain all seriously ill people would second mortgage their homes, beg, borrow or steal to try the big thing he was offering. Even I spent the last of my retirement money to try his "big thing". That's when I came full circle to the truth of what Bud Curtis said over 30 years ago: All the expensive and even good therapies in the world can't heal you if you don't *first* remove the thorn.

Indeed, what I've found is that many nutrients and therapies can be beneficial to alleviate symptoms or *help* the body heal — *but* the path to complete or near complete freedom from disease and pain is not so much what you do, but what you don't do (although some diseases involve a level of damage so severe that complete reversal may only be hoped for by the application of stem cells). In fact, with regard to healing, recently "Dr. Oz" on Oprah stated something that I've known from my own body, but is contrary to what medicine has taught for decades. He said that we've previously held the belief that only certain organs can repair and regenerate. Here it is, this is BIG: **"We now know that *all* cells, tissues and organs can repair and regenerate."** (Again, some tissues can be so damaged, like brain damage from an accident, or kidney damage from toxins, that it would involve the addition of stem cells for a complete healing).

Speaking of stem cells, it's only been since the year 2000, that the floodgates have opened on the understanding about our body's own lifetime production of stem cells (mostly in the bone marrow). Prior to 2000 all the general public knew about stem cells was basically that the government was fighting research on embryonic stem cells. I, too, thought that once an organ like your kidneys or brain was damaged, there could be no healing. But I discovered differently after finding my own kidney tests improving (from only 50-60% function to 70-80%) after using stem cell enhancing supplements and avoiding analgesics (the pain-killers were the "thorn").

There has been for decades, and still exists to a great degree, the erroneous conviction by the medical profession, that "once damaged always damaged". This is tragic because when people find out they have cancer or kidney disease or even a tooth that feels like it needs a root canal — they *rush* to the doctor, trusting the doctor to fix the problem.

Because all the doctor has in his tool box are drugs, radiation and surgery, the poor person ends up poisoning their body with the toxic drugs, burning themselves with the radiation or completely losing the "offending" body part. How *should* we handle the diagnosis? First alleviate the pain – then work to *discern the true underlying cause of the problem*. Then apply every detox method and healing modality to allow the body to *heal* the diseased body part. The body does this far better than man because while healing the one body part, the entire body is also healing. This scenario is not being played out, however. People are not *removing* the thorn, but are adding more thorns!

Indeed, there is a critical and immediate need for everyone, and especially "health care providers" to wake up to truths of which they are either currently ignorant or *choose to ignore* because the truth is inconvenient or contrary to what they were formerly taught or believed. I have learned that many people who earn money in the "health care field" fear that the truth won't generate the kind of money they want to make. I myself have gone like a lamb to slaughter to people who advertise as "holistic", "alternative", "nutritional" and been recommended and given costly procedures that were unnecessary and even furthered my disease and pain process. I've lost track after $90,000 that I've spent completely out of pocket in just the last 6 years. I can't get that money back, and I have gotten very little in return for it.

There Are Truths *Most* People Just Don't Know

Since breaking out from head to toe with psoraisis at the age of 11, I've embarked on over 40 years that now at age 54, has taught me the following (all of which becomes clearer throughout this entire book):

I. Our government is *allowing* poisons like glutamates and mercury in our food supply and medicines. There are so many poisons, in fact, that they are now "household words", and virtually ignored by the average consumer, even though they are *causing* our devastating diseases! For example – we have found an alarming number of imports from China to be tainted with lead – are you *still* buying things from China? Lead is so toxic an 8-year old girl accidentally swallowed a little bracelet from China – and died. A little boy swallowed a little "silver" heart charm given to him when his mother bought him some athletic shoes. No-one knew he had swallowed it. After his death it was found in his intestines and analyzed. It was nearly pure lead. So *why* are you still buying things from China? Likely your unconcern is because "nobody seems alarmed". And "nobody" (meaning governing agencies) don't show alarm partly as a coverup, which is enormous and calculated (to prevent massive lawsuits as well as prevent complete distrust in the government agencies that are supposed to be watchdogs protecting us). Indeed, if the word "coverup" makes you think I'm being an "alarmist" – you haven't been doing your homework. Actually, the "coverup" is quite exposed (you only need to look) in thousands of scientific studies, lawsuits and pending lawsuits, news stories, as well as millions of parents who suspect or even *know* that mercury is, indeed, the underlying cause of their child's autism, Tourette's Syndrome, ADD, epilepsy, multiple sclerosis, etc. Much of this is swept under political rugs.

2. When you get sick, and go to the doctor, doctors are *clueless* as to what *caused* the disease in the first place. A doctor's first thought is to merely ameliorate symptoms, and worse…recommend very dangerous drugs, radiation, surgeries that in the end, *don't work* and are causing far more suffering and death than they purport to ameliorate. I heard a doctor tell a talk show host just recently (2008) talking about someone with cancer: "We know we can't get the patient well, so we give them all kinds of tests, therapies, drugs and surgeries…so at least they *feel* like we're really "doing something". (What?? Is he thinking out loud? It's the truth, but did he mean to spill the beans? Think what this means about the trillions that are spent on "healthcare" each year.) Indeed, if doctors could heal people, they would say "heal", not "in remission". It won't be until you eliminate the

underlying cause of a disease, and apply true healing therapies, like complete dietary and lifestyle changes and stem
cells that true *healing* can occur.

3. When doctors can't help you and you've gone to them half a
dozen times for the same thing only to be sent home to suffer, insurance companies then refuse to cover you. So we end
up with millions of sick Americans without insurance. This
leads to entire families losing their savings, their homes, and
their very security from huge "medical" costs (that don't even
work!) *It's true.* I applied for insurance recently (2007) and
was told, "You went to the doctor three or more times last
year. Sorry, you'll have to inquire about "high risk" insurance." When I inquired about high risk insurance the cost
was $700-1400 a month. I could either have a roof over my
head, or health insurance that I didn't really even want because
no doctor has ever helped me (but insurance I *needed* in case
of an accident or poisoning or something). It's bad enough
that emergency rooms are closing because of people who
are unable to pay for the services. Now we have hard-work-
ing Americans without the insurance security blanket they
deserve.

4. The good news is that if you don't damage yourself too badly
trying this drug or that surgery first, *God's medicines work to heal-*
where man's medicines most often ultimately cause more damage and more disease. If you don't "believe" in God, simply
substitute "Nature" where I say God. I know unequivocally
that God's medicines work with your own powerful healing
mechanisms of antioxidant protectors, enzyme facilitators,
hormone orchestrators, stem cell rebuilders and more. Everything a human body needs to heal is both within your own
body and on this earth in Nature – if *you don't get in the way*
by damaging yourself irreversibly first. God's medicines include
organic, whole foods (God-given state – nothing added, nothing taken away); herbs; sunshine; pure water; fresh air (oxygen); activity/exercise – *and above all – avoidance and removal of*
"thorns"!

My Own Health History

I was born the 6th child (my brother, the 7th and last, came four years later) in Whittier, California. I spent my first dozen years in La Mirada, California. In La Mirada I remember being a fairly normal child health-wise. My "health memories" are of the "normal" childhood diseases like mumps, measles and such. I was never rushed to the emergency room needing tubes in my ears. Neither did I get any of the diseases that start in childhood today, and are truly epidemic, like asthma, ADD, autism, epilepsy and diabetes.

Indeed, I remember feeling good and playing outside most of the day, every day. The only odd health memory were frequent **hives**. I recall never being taken to the doctor, but when I didn't feel well, I just went to bed. The closest I came to a doctor was a neighbor dad who sold pharmaceuticals. Once when I stupidly jumped down from a bathroom sink and cut myself right between the legs on the open cabinet below (yep…in the privates), my mother called that neighbor dad to "take a look at it". I was mortified!

We moved from La Mirada to San Clemente when I was 11. My father now owned a Schwinn bicycle franchise, but was also a raging alcoholic. We bought a beautiful ocean-view home and managed to keep it until after my parents split up when I was out of high school. It was there in San Clemente where my life changed *most* drastically that first year, age 11, when for perhaps only the second or third time in my life I went to a dentist. But this time I was told I had 8 cavities. Within a week or two I walked out of that dental office with 8 shiny new silver-colored amalgam fillings. Within just months I was covered from head to toe with psoriasis – nasty, thick, ugly plaques on my skin and scalp. (See Chapter 7 *Psoriasis*).

It was at this same time, age 11, 7th grade, I vividly recall a very unusual thing that would happen as I played on the playground. This was after the amalgams, and after the psoriasis (which was worse in 7th and 8th grade than ever because I didn't have a clue how to deal with the psoriasis). I remember bouncing a ball in the "Four Square" game out on the playground, or hitting a tetherball around the pole, and suddenly I would experience a hot "POP" deep in my brain on the right side – as if a blood vessel had exploded or "cramped". It happened frequently, perhaps two to three times per week…but I'd forgotten all about it until recently. I remember I would stop what I was doing, frightened, waiting to see if something worse was going to happen. It seemed to pass, left me shaken, and I would carry on with my day. This continued into my teens, and then it must have abated, as I don't recall it happening anymore past high school. Remember this when you read Chapter 8 *Migraines*.

Psoriasis went on to ruin my teen years. While other teens were dating, going to the beach, going on camping trips, joining the swim team, getting fancy hair-dos for the "Prom", I hid. There would be no putting my hair up to reveal large thick lesions of nasty psoriasis. In fact, once when visiting my aunt, I'd put my hair up to lay out in the sun (which I discovered helped keep my psoriasis under control) but she pointed to the thick patches behind my ear and made some juvenile comment about it being nasty.

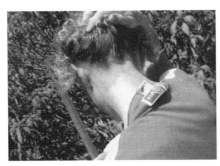 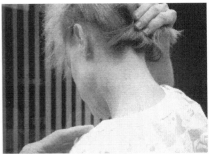

Psoriasis before I knew what to do – huge patches of redness and scales

Psoriasis after I knew what to do – *there are no patches of redness and scales here*

Of course, the ugliness and "shame" of it is exactly why I "hid" as much as possible (but you'd think an adult would know better than to comment). I felt like a leper. I planned my life around the sun. I wouldn't get a job in the daytime because I needed to lay out in the sun to keep my psoriasis under control. No amount of topicals (like Tegrin) did more than make me smell bad. I soaked in the tub to remove scales, and lay in the sun to heal the redness underneath. It was a full-time job in itself.

I did manage to go to college, however I didn't finish in four years, it took about twelve. I was unsettled and handicapped by the psoriasis. At one time I thought, "Should I be a nurse?" I knew I wanted to help people. But I couldn't pull my hair up like nurses did for fear of revealing that ugly psoriasis. This haunted me for decades, until I went back to try to enroll in nursing school in my forties. But it was too late – I was too busy with family and too "old" to go to school with the intensity that would be required. But it wasn't meant to be anyway. I had already graduated with a Bachelor of Science degree years prior. I had also earned my certification as a nutritionist. I was meant to do something else.

Setting About To Remove Those Thorns

During about a 6 year period before I was married, there was a time when, in my mid-twenties, still going to college, I'd lost a lot of weight and my lymph glands were swollen. I found a "nutritionally-oriented" doctor, because by now I knew that the usual "allopathic" doctors didn't have any answers for me. I'd been to a few for the psoriasis and all they had to offer was ineffective and even dangerous salves and medications. One cortisone ointment I tried caused a horrific fungal overgrowth!

It was at this time a "nutritionally-oriented" doctor did some tests and upon a return visit called his colleague into the room. They openly discussed that I had "lymphoma". They wanted to do some further invasive procedures but I wouldn't let them. Angrily, he dismissed me and told me he thought I'd be dead in 6-9 months.

My soon-to-be husband drove me home, crying. I told him not to worry – I had a plan. Indeed, I knew what had to be done – and it wasn't drugs, radiation or surgery. I immediately embarked upon what would be approximately 12 years going to various health clinics and resorts and eating only whole, raw, organic foods. God's medicines. I ate sprouts and drank and did wheatgrass implants at the Optimum Health Institute. I had an iridological exam by Bernard Jensen and stayed at Hidden Valley Health Ranch. I underwent polarity therapy and ate all vegetarian at Dr. Loomis' in Hemet. I did coffee enemas and drank raw liver juice at Max Gerson's in Mexico. I did intravenous hydrogen peroxide therapies at Jimmy Keller's in Tijuana and then also at home. I drove out into the desert to meet Bud Curtis and learn about his ozone therapies. I got sun and sweated, I walked and bicycled. I purified the water I drank as well as the household air. I did the best I could do to detoxify and rebuild at the cellular level – and it worked. My lymph glands were my barometer and they kept getting smaller and smaller and I regained all my weight.

But life went on during these 12 years. While it was obvious that I was getting well within just a year or two, I kept doing all the raw foods and various therapies for about 12 years until the very last lymph gland went down to normal size. That I'm here is proof it worked, of course, but the main reason it worked (I hope all healthcare practitioners are listening) is not as much because of what I did, but what I _didn't_ do. I didn't cut, burn or poison myself (surgery, radiation, drugs). My body was given a chance to heal, and because of that I'm here still today with no sign of lymphoma. I did have a couple of reoccurence scares many years ago when I let my guard down (glands seemed to be enlarging), but I returned to raw foods, and added new things I learned along the way, like "Car-T-Cell" a preparation of shark cartilage some studies have shown counteracts cancer.

I had my wisdom teeth removed in my late 20's but I didn't have it done the way I now know it should be (see Chapter 6 _Dental Work_). Shortly thereafter I began having **headaches** which were worse during my last two pregnancies. I worried, in fact, that all of the Tylenol I was taking would harm my baby (thankfully it didn't).

In my early 30's while working at a childcare facility when my second child (my son) was about 2 or 3, I remember a sensation in my brain as if there was a "marble" in there putting pressure or exerting a gaseous "bubbling" effect. Recall the playground incidence when I was only 11 – when there was a hot "popping" sensation – this "marble" was in the exact same spot. I would sit out on the grass watching the kids play, pulling on my hair on the right side of my head as if to pull that marble out. This went on for a few years. Because I thought I might have a brain tumor, I went to a health spa where wheatgrass was the primary therapy. After drinking wheatgrass juice and doing "implants" for several weeks I was awakened from a sound sleep with a "pop" in that area of my brain. This wasn't a "hot" pop – but more of a release. The sensation of bubbling and pressure ceased. But more than 20 years of migraines later I now know that the "bubbling" was occuring where a Tesla MRI now shows I have "white matter lesions" (see Chapter 9 *Multiple Sclerosis* for photo of the MRI).

A Botched Epidural

I'd given birth to my son (second child) when I was 31 and during labor an anesthesiologist tried to give me an epidural to ease my labor pains. It was completely botched. He was a cocky young resident who waltzed into the room where I had been laboring unproductively for over 12 hours. He told the nurses, "watch how fast I can do this". In case you don't know, an epidural uses a catheter needle, and it's much larger than the "hair-thin" needle doctors use right into the spine for a "spinal". The anesthesiologist needs to slowly push this catheter needle into the back and feel the layers surrounding the spine to get only into the epidurum, and not the spine itself. One doctor later told me it's four layers into the spine, and that the doctor's job is to stop short of that fourth layer. But this cocky young resident didn't. He was trying to impress the nurses and do the job "quickly" causing him to go right into the spine with a large hole he now had created. He didn't realize his error yet, though, as he told me my legs would feel numb in about 15-20 minutes. But they were numb instantly. He looked shocked, said no more, and quickly left the room.

Well, I gave birth to my son with the epidural catheter still in my back. The protocol calls for it's removal after the birth. But it was left in for many hours. Later when they removed it, WHAM! I suffered a headache unlike any I'd ever had, with violent nausea. The pain and nausea was greater than a 10 on the scale of pain. I laid in the hospital bed for 4 days in agony – begging God to take me. I remember nurses would bring me my baby and I didn't know if it was a boy or a girl. They'd scold me and tell me I needed to "get up and take care of the baby". But I was horribly nauseous and in debilitating pain. Then on the fourth day a senior anesthesiologist, a woman, came into my room and told me a hole had been created when the catheter was removed and my meningeal fluid had "drained" from the protective meningeal lining around my spine and brain. That, she said, is what was causing the horrific "headache" and nausea. She said I had to sign a release to give them permission to withdraw blood from my arm and then find the exact hole and inject the blood so it would coagulate, closing up the hole, allowing the meningeal fluid to stay put. She told me it could go one of two ways. I'd either sit up instantly and the headache would be gone – and I could go home...or they'd miss the hole and I'd be paralyzed. What an option! But frankly, at that point I didn't care. I signed. Then a shock! In came that young anesthesiologist. The hospital was going to make him "fix" what he'd "broken"! Again, I wanted to die anyway...so I didn't put up a fight. Well, obviously he was successful. But that was the beginning of my chronic migraines!

Today I believe that the draining of the protective meningeal fluid that is part of the blood-brain barrier finished a job that had started with mercury damage to my brain. It could be that my dormant herpes virus had easy access when my defenses were down during that 4 day period of a "hole" in my armor, and lives today along the trigeminal nerve up to where mercury has damaged my brain. I've had the herpes I, herpes II and herpes zoster symptoms and outbreaks in many places all over my body before that incidence – it's a matter of where you're left defenseless or where you're damaged. Parasites like herpes are opportunistic. It could also be that during that period there was mercury in some of the medicines I was being given, and they were doing even further damage to my brain. But it all started with the popping in my brain after having those amalgams (mercury) placed in my teeth as an 11 year old.

About this same time of giving birth to my second child, I was working for Dr. Julian Whitaker in Newport Beach. This partnership would continue for over 15 years. At first I planned and cooked the meals for the live-in program. I did this for years. At the same time I helped him write his first four books and a cookbook. I gave nutrition lectures to his patients during their two week stay at his live-in program. I became his corporate comptroller. I helped him design his large new facility. It was a job made in Heaven for me. After I left that job I worked for a nutritionally-oriented chiropractor for 5 years, then a holistic D.O. for whom I still research and write as of 2008. All the while my headaches continued and worsened in severity and frequency. I was in search of answers.

From Headaches to Migraines

My headaches continued, and worsened during my third pregnancy. Then, after my third child the terrible headaches went deeper into the brain and became full-blown migraines. I have to say, it is my experience that most people have no clue what a migraine really is. It's not a headache. In fact, when I hear that someone got Botox shots in the muscle of their neck or temple and they no longer have migraines, with what I know, there's no way that person had true migraines. Perhaps they had cluster headache or tension headache - but likely not migraines. You can't "paralyze" a muscle to get rid of what is occuring deep within the brain.

Migraines are a neurological firestorm (See Chapter 8 *Migraines*) that occur very deep in the brain. Anyone who has had any pain involving the nerves knows that the pain is excrutiating and the kind of pain that makes you beg to die. Couple that with the fact that many migraines are accompanied by nausea, and you end up with pain in the "worst pain on earth" category. In fact, I saw a book recently rating various types of pain, and migraines were right up there with bone cancer – both rated a "10" on a scale of 1-10. Of course the bone cancer is continuous and far worse than "a migraine" which eventually ends. But while it is occuring a migraine is beyond unbearable, *especially* when accompanied by nausea. No wonder some news stories about migraines show a sufferer literally banging their head on the ground, and crawling to the bathroom to vomit time and time again.

Describing a Migraine

I have tried to describe my own migraine pain many times but couldn't remember well enough in-between migraines – thankfully we humans have a built-in "forget" mechanism when it comes to physical pain. So one time while I was having a migraine I forced myself to sit down and write how it felt:

"It is as if half of your brain is on fire and brain matter is black and smoldering, with a sickening smell and toxic gasses rising from the charred embers. But these toxic gasses have no where to go, and so are infiltrating the other side of your brain, your eyes, your neck, down into your entire body. You can feel the sick, syrupy warmth deep inside your brain. You're nauseated all over. But there's no relief. You can't just rub your temples, because that's not where the pain is. The pain eminates from deep in the brain. The pain is excrutiating." Now multiply the pain you are imagining times ten.

Mercury Caused My Migraines

Again, I trace my migraines back to when, at the age of 11, I had 8 amalgam fillings placed. The "popping" in my head on the right side shortly thereafter was the precursor damage to my migraines. Then, in my early 30's when the protective layer of my brain, the meningeal fluid, was literally "drained" my brain was left unprotected and further damage was done. Mercury from amalgams had already laid the groundwork damaging the glutamatergic system (the amino acid transporter cells that "recycle" glutamate) and immune system (See Chapter 3 *Pollutants* and Chapter 8 *Migraines*). In fact, a recent Tesla MRI showed that I have white matter lesions – damage – exactly in the spot where my migraines eminate. The white matter lesions are also right where I felt the pressure and "bubbling" about 3 years before the full-blown migraines began. The herpes zoster virus that resides dormant along nerves, resides along my trigeminal nerve which goes up into my brain and down the side of my face and jaw. I've now had "trigeminal neuralgia" which I know is from that herpes virus (because efforts to fight the virus stopped the horrific pain when nothing else would - *including an unnecessary root canal!*)

Had there never been any mercury, there would never have been any migraines, trigeminal neuralgia, and so much suffering.

> When the health effects of **mercury** were investigated, the most frequently observed symptom was cephalalgia (**headaches**). [*Biol Trace Elem Res* 2002 Winter;90(1-3):1-14.]

The researchers in the above-quoted study suggested that metals might be introduced as possible biological markers for the diagnosis and therapy of different headache syndromes in future clinical trials and laboratory measurements. That was in 2002. I could find no studies doing any such thing from then until now. I'm still looking.

Coping With Migraines

In the 1980's I learned about the aforementioned Dr. Max Gerson who developed a successful program for cancer, when quite by accident, as he was trying to deal with his own migraines, he discovered the coffee enema. I embarked on over 10 years of doing coffee enemas to get rid of a migraine. In the early years it worked about 80% of the time. The caffeine in the coffee, I learned, goes up the portal vein to the liver where it stimulates the bile ducts to open and dump their toxins. That's why he used it for cancer. But for migraines, dumping the liver toxins helps to take away nausea. But I think the action is mostly due to the fact that the caffeine travels in the bloodstream throughout the vasculature where it acts as a vasoconstrictor on veins that are dilated as a part of the migraine "syndrome". When the veins constrict, at least 80% of the time the pain will go away. For most of my migraines this worked like a charm. As the years went by, and estrogen (hormonal migraines) became involved, *nothing* would work...not coffee enemas, and not even "Excedrin for Migraines".

In the mid-80's I became more aware of the amalgam-mercury issue. But it still wasn't something most people had heard of. With the pain of migraines as my motivator, I travelled to a dentist an hour away (Santa Monica) to have all my amalgams removed. This was a woman dentist who knew mercury was bad, but had no clue how to take it out properly. In *one sitting* all the amalgams were removed (I had about 10), composite fillings were placed, and I was prepped for about 4 gold crowns. *Wrong.* I drove home sicker than a dog. I was nauseous. I had a horrific migraine. I vomited. When I got home I did about 4 coffee enemas in a row...they didn't help. I suffered horribly. This went on for two days. I finally got over the migraine...but the mercury vapors contributed to a worsening of my diseases, and more pain. I know this, because my migraines didn't go away – and actually worsened. So, at the time I thought the mercury removal "did nothing" (I didn't realize it had actually done more harm) and turned my attention again to other things like diet and supplements.

In June of 2003 after years of once to twice monthly migraines (that's every other week!) where so often I couldn't attend a wedding or party or go to a job – I decided to look into migraine medications. I did some research, called on a family member who had had success with medications, and then made an appointment with a doctor. He prescribed Imitrex for me. This Imitrex experiment was horrific from day one. I got the injectible kind because of how quickly it worked. The first shot was frightening, as was the second and every shot I injected thereafter. It felt like I had been shocked with defibrillator paddles. I had to lay down. My heart raced. I prayed for God to not let me die from the medicine. But the migraine and nausea were gone within minutes.

I continued to use the Imitrex until September of that year. But I needed it more and more, yet was allowed only 9 shots per month (at over $100.00 a shot!). With my background in alternative, herbal and natural methods, the entire experience was disconcerting to say the least. But then one September morning I got into my car and reached back for my seatbelt, and it felt as if someone had shot me in the shoulder with a gun. That excrutiatingly painful incident initiated 11 months of lupus-like symptoms: Bones that ached horribly, a butterfly rash across my nose, depression, weakness, difficulty getting enough oxygen. At the time I was also observing a friend who was taking an even stronger form of migraine medicine called Frova (a triptan like Imitrex). After taking Frova she's had surgery on her neck, her back always hurts, she seemed to be encountering one health problem after another. She, too, had found that nine doses per month was not enough. Needless to say, I stopped the Imitrex immediately. It took 11 months for my lupus-like symptoms to abate. I couldn't reach up or behind my back at all (like to button or zipper or to set my hair) it was so painful, and I was so weak. I couldn't even reach my left arm up to wash my hair without excrutiating pain. I thought, "you've really done it this time!"

Then Multiple Sclerosis

Then in 2004, after the lupus-like symptoms finally seemed a thing of the past, I started an Esthetician course with my 16 year old daughter, hoping to be right there to help her get through it and graduate (and she did). At the end of the year-long course, it was recommended that we get hepatitis shots because of working closely with people. I had been of the "Esthetician" mindset for a year, and not the health researcher mindset. I stupidly thought, "it's just a dead virus, isn't it?" The school had scared me into wanting to get the shots. I had the hepatitis A shot first and nothing happened out of the ordinary. A few weeks later I went for the hepatitis B shot. Within hours I had twitching down the radial nerve on the arm along where the shot had been given. This twitching lasted for weeks and nearly drove me crazy. As it subsided, symptoms like multiple sclerosis began. I had complete numbness in my fingers and feet. I even had numbness along the calves of my legs and up my arms. I would get up in the night to go to the bathroom and my legs felt wooden and heavy. I had "restless leg syndrome" that kept me up until 3 and 4 in the morning. Then the cramping - the horrific, "I want to die" cramping in my feet, hands, arms and legs. It was unbearable. I won't bore you with the details, just that there were many other symptoms, not the least of which were "waves" of depression where I'd be in a room with the people I loved most, even doing what I loved most (playing games, or music) and I felt utter despair - a horrible feeling that has now taught me what true depression is.

Well, I did my research quickly and found Calcium AEP. This was studied extensively in Germany and found to alleviate those neurological symptoms. I found the best product at Vitamin Research Products in vegetarian capsules and bought many bottles. I started taking it right away – *immediately and still now, 4 years later, all the symptoms are kept under control if I take enough CaAEP.* While I've had to increase the dose as the years have gone by, I know that people taking a drug would have to take an entire bottle of a supplement to even come close to the "danger" of the drug. I now take about 8-10 capsules per day. I think of diabetics who have to "monitor their insulin", taking from 1 unit daily to many units daily depending upon their blood glucose levels. It's no different with CaAEP, except that this is a natural supplement, and you'd likely have to take an entire bottle of it daily every day for many years to even begin to show any signs of anything approaching excess. With supplements, simply stopping the supplement should return your body to its previous state. Not so with drugs, which can do permanent, even deadly damage.

I am also, of course, doing many other things, for example, I will never again submit to amalgams or vaccinations or any other heavy metal sources knowingly. (See more information in Chapter 11 – *Nature's Medicines*)

What Caused The Psoriasis, Migraines & MS?

There is absolutely, positively no question – the psoriais, migraines, MS – *were all caused by mercury* (See Chapter 5 *All The Things Going On*). Where did I get the mercury? Well, what you may not know is that in spite of the propaganda, even in 2004, vaccines *still* contained mercury. The hepatitis B vaccine, for some reason contained a whopping 12.5 mcg. Then, in 2006, my precious granddaughter was born. I was there. Just in the nick of time I stopped a nurse from injecting that newborn baby with a hepatitis B vaccine! I asked her if there was mercury in it. She looked at the label and said, "just a trace". I told her *mercury is highly toxic - even a trace!* I never allowed my three, now adult, children to be vaccinated, nor did I allow them to have silver (mercury) fillings. Neither has my precious granddaughter had vaccines, and all four are free of any of the chronic and debilitating diseases that "everybody" has one or more of these days.

And That Isn't All

Throughout the years struggling with psoriasis, suffering horribly from migraines, the eleven year journey with lymphoma, and now multiple sclerosis - I suffered from one herpes outbreak after another, pneumonia, ulcers, a bout of trigemnial neuralgia, pleurisy and many other types of issues or infections. Since age 11 and eight mercury fillings, my immune system has been *shot*. I know now it's all due to mercury, but my mother will tell you she worried she didn't have time to recuperate to give me the best possible chance for optimum health. I was born in 1953, and my brother before me, in 1952. No, I was born perfectly healthy, and lived the first ten years of my life in quite good health. Mercury has been the thorn in my life.

The truth is we *all* have or know someone who has these various health issues. In fact, having many "health issues" is so commonplace, many now believe it is *normal*, but it most certainly is not. The people who suffer daily *know* it isn't "normal".

That said, I sat rather impatiently just last night through yet another Oprah/Dr. Oz episode (and I like Dr. Oz just fine). This episode was about his book "You: The Owner's Manual". As my husband watched with rapt attention, making comments of agreement, I couldn't believe my ears. After all these years of my proving that *pollutants* + *parasites* are causing our epidemic of diseases, pain, and *aging*...my own sweet husband was buying into the same wrong emphasis on diet, exercise, stress, etc. Dr. Oz had an "announcement" – the "number one" cause of aging. After the commerical here it was: *Stress*. Now, he meant the kind of stress we're all "feeling" because of such a hectic schedule. "Bull!" Stress didn't cause my psoriasis, mercury did. Stress didn't cause my migraines, mercury did. Stress didn't cause my MS, mercury did. Stress isn't good, of course, but it's something man has had to endure since prehistoric times. No, stress doesn't continue to pommel our bodies into further disease and pain – *pollutants and parasites do.* Do the right diet, calming techniques, exercises, etc. help? Of course. The problem is this: If the belief is that "stress" is the underlying *cause* of your disease – you will continue to walk blindly down a dark tunnel leading to a hellish experience on earth experiencing chronic disease, pain, and financial ruin. Now that's stress!

Do you know that in the entire program, Dr. Oz didn't even mention mercury, pesticides, free glutamates, or even smoking as a "number one" cause of anything! Yet smoking statistically kills more people every year than *any other single thing!* He also didn't even utter the word "virus" or bacteria or fungus - not once. Again, as my husband sat "eating it all up" I was incredulous that my husband, whose been fed all the right information – that even *he* could be beguiled by this baloney.

So *why* do people buy into this nonsense? A conclusion I'd come to prior to ever watching Dr. Oz is that "diet", "exercise", "stress reduction" – are all "glamorous" and understandable and within the "reach" of people who are suffering. *No one* wants to believe they've been poisoned – much less that they are continuing to be poisoned. By what? When? Where? What can I do? I have to do *what???* Pull out some teeth? Move? Not use my cell phone? That's all too difficult. Can't I just include cruciferous vegetables daily in my diet or do yoga? Now we're back to feeling more in control.

Beginning Glimpses Of Truth

The very first thing I ever read about psoriasis was in a health book I'd stumbled upon as a 13 year old. That book said that psoriasis is as a result of being "dirty" inside. Ouch! People also don't want to think of themselves as dirty inside! This is why people don't cozy up to the word "parasite", but prefer bacteria, virus and even "candida" over fungus! However, there is truth to the "dirty" inside notion. Of course *mercury* initially causes immune damage, which allows the overgrowth of candida, and gut damage that actually causes a person to be "dirty inside" and their body to end up with the symptom of psoriasis. In fact, Candida is one parasite growing in *many* people (not just psoriatics) resulting in "dirty" gut resulting in "dirty" blood (See Chapter 7 *Psoriasis*). The other side of the coin is something I read as a child that has also stayed with me ever since: "When you're green inside, you're clean inside." There's volumes of truth to that, as well. (See Chapter 11 *Nature's Medicines*).

No Pollutants = No Disease = No Pain

I hope to make it crystal clear that if there were no pollutants, our bodies would rarely succumb to opportunistic parasites, and there would be little to no disease or pain. Truly — we would all die of old age — not disease. Even the worst parasites are meant to be handled by a strong immune system, undamaged by pollutants. Of course we'd want to work to eradicate any known parasites as even the strongest immune system would succumb if attacked too long by too many. Nevertheless, pollutants are *clearly* the initial destructive force in *all* diseases, after which opportunistic parasites can invade and do their dirty work. I also hope to make it clear that man's medicines simply don't work most of the time, *especially* when your doctor can't tell you *exactly* what caused your disease. "Practicing" in medicine has got to stop. I've experienced firsthand the damage done by doctors "trying" various drugs on me. In fact, if I solicited the stories of others, I believe I could fill an entire encyclopedia of books with drug horror stories.

On the other hand, I have experienced firsthand that God's medicines can work to truly heal. By God's medicines, I mean first and foremost *removing* pollutants, but also consuming foods free of poisons (like pesticides and excitotoxins), as well as using herbs, sunshine, and activity, as God intended. The only reason anyone would think that's God's ways aren't best, is because they didn't do the research to discern the underlying *cause* of their disease(s) so they continue, literally, to poison themselves! One example is if you get a flu shot year after year (contains mercury) then not knowing why you are sinking deeper and deeper into a neurological disease. Mercury is the number one perpetrator of all neurological diseases.

Not only that, but *flu shots don't work!* (See section *The Rabbit* where Dr. Mercola called a vaccine company, and they admitted the flu shots don't even work).

What do you do to not get the flu? Consume *no dairy*, especially during flu season. Dairy produces the perfect mucous environment for infections to proliferate. Also take care to consume copious organic raw fruits and vegetables as well as taking supplemental vitamin C and zinc as these stave off a cold or flu, and should stop either dead in its tracks should they occur. In addition there are immune-enhancing supplements outlined in Chapter 11 *Nature's Medicines* that should be taken around the clock when the first signs of a cold or flu or any infection occurs.

> Two years ago a study in the *British Medical Journal* concluded that the effectiveness of annual **flu shots** has been exaggerated, and that in reality they have little or no effect...Other studies, done prior and subsequently, also confirm these findings. However, preventing flu-related deaths in the elderly has been, and still is, the primary argument for recommending flu shots each year...the flu prevention strategy set by the Centers for Disease Control and Prevention (CDC) has been called into serious question time and again. Another study from 2005, published in the *Archives of Internal Medicine* also could not find support for the use of flu vaccine to prevent deaths in the elderly. The report highlights that although immunization rates in people over 65 have increased dramatically in the past 20 years, **there has not been a consequent decline in flu-related deaths.** (See entire report as well as a phone call to flu vaccine manufacturer who admits there is *still* mercury in the flu vaccine *and that even vaccines claiming they have no "thimerosal" contain traces of mercury!*) [http://articles.mercola.com/sites/articles/archive/2008/11/18/do-flu-shots-work-ask-a-vaccine-manufacturer.aspx]

Flu shots have contained mercury for decades, and as of this year, the multi-use vials can still contain mercury. Note that on the cover of this book is a photo of healthy neurons. In Chapter 9 *Multiple Sclerosis*, is a photo of a neuron before and after being exposed to the tiniest bit of mercury. The neuron is completely damaged. Keep in mind that **the researchers then challenged neurons with other metals like aluminum and lead** *but these did not damage the neuron like mercury did.*

40+ Years Of Fighting, Still Going Strong

Knowing the truth starts with *wanting* to know the truth. I've sought the truth for over 40 years of my life out of necessity. Pain is a real motivator. I understand that without pain most people simply aren't motivated – even when they have a terrible disease! I've also learned that most people find comfort in having a team of medical people hustling and bustling around, reassuring them not to worry, "your insurance will cover this" – even if *"this"* won't work, and will likely harm them even more!

I've learned firsthand, that even when you know exactly what to do, and what not to do, as a human being you'll always try to see how far you can push the envelope. "Can't" eat dairy? Because you love frozen yogurt, you'll see just how many times you can eat it before you suffer the ill effects. Is it once a week? Once a month? I'm no different. I sometimes "cheat". But as new alarming and painful symptoms have popped up such as when I didn't have any idea an "innocent" vaccine had 12.5 mcg of poison in it – comes yet another resolve for the truth, and nothing but the truth.

So this book tells you what I've learned about mercury, about root canals, about the actual cause of migraines versus "all the things going on", about multiple sclerosis and so much more. I share my own experiences, but mostly something most people don't have access to or understand – the studies, the lawsuits, the documentations, the quotes that are your thousands of puzzle pieces, that when put together make a very clear picture: **Pollutants** (and with neurological diseases, first is mercury) *caused* your disease. **Parasites** are opportunistic and come along to dine on your diseased cells like vultures.

So That's My 40+ Years In A Nutshell

That's where I'm at folks. If you aren't suffering yourself, you likely cannot fully understand. I'm documenting these amazing, alarming, life-changing, shocking (all that and more) truths in this book, because when you *do* want the information — likely because you're in chronic pain, or someone you love is in chronic pain — what I have to offer will be there for you, so you (or they) won't have to waste half a lifetime searching for answers while suffering, and perhaps coming up emptyhanded.

The important points you need to understand, and the entire purpose of this book:

- *Mercury* is the number one culprit causing damage to everyone's body by the simple fact that everyone is being injected with, eating and having it placed permanently in their mouths
- Just one area of damage by mercury is damage to the *gluta-matergic system* i.e., that system that activates the synapsing of neurons, and thus the proper functioning of everything in the body
- A damaged glutamatergic system creates *excess glutamates* and is unable to properly utilize, break down, recycle and eliminate glutamate
- The excess glutamates cause ongoing damage (like death to neurons and the protective coating around them) as well as fueling excess *inflammatory compounds* like CGRP, Substance P and nitric oxide
- Nitric Oxide in excess causes the extreme *vasodilatation* seen in migraines and other inflammatory conditions
- *Parasites* like herpes feast on diseased cells like vultures
- *Deficiencies* leave your cells defenseless. There are thousands upon thousands of God-made nutrients that are absolutely necessary to protect your cells from damage and death — and can only be gotten from a diet made up nearly entirely of pure, fresh, whole, (preferably organic) mostly raw, plant foods

Chapter 2
ONE OUT OF TWO PEOPLE GETTING
A DEVASTATING DISEASE

I did some research through many organizations online that list how many people have certain diseases. If you Google "Disease Statistics" you will come up with government sites like the Center For Disease Control (CDC). After many hours pouring over the various diseases on various sites, I added up the numbers and found that of our current 303 million population in America (2008), *at least* **161.5 million have one of many life-robbing, life-threatening, life-shortening diseases** (see below) – some of which are "death sentences", others that alter your life completely, and others that can lead to worse diseases – but certainly take their toll financially, physically and emotionally. Consider also there are *dozens* of other diseases I don't even list. In listing just those that I do, we see there are more than 53% of the population with a serious illness that goes on to *ruin* their life, their finances, precious time with loved ones, and their joy. Indeed, if you add up the statistics....over 5 million with Alzheimer's, etc. and compare that to the overall population, the statistics tell the story: 53% of the population (age doesn't matter) have a serious illness....about one in two. This is because every other person has "something". As I mentioned previously, I know of a 10 year old with Parkinson's. So if it seems unbelievable that people under 40 are now coming down with what *used* to be considered "elderly" diseases – go ahead and be astounded, but it's true.

These figures are actually *conservative.* Consider migraines. They are not on this list, but devastating in pain, loss of days, loss of joy, and financial ruin – *and* they can lead to or are associated with worse diseases, like strokes and multiple sclerosis. Speaking of multiple sclerosis there are many people who have it, but because it is costly and difficult to diagnose, are under the radar of the folks that put these statistics together, so they're not included in the 40,000 on this list. The truth about how many people have a devastating disease is, in my opinion and experience, approaching more like 2 in 3 or 66%.

Disease	How Many People Have It
ALZHEIMER'S	Over 5 million are thought to have Alzheimer's with 65,829 deaths per year
ALS Amyotrophic Lateral Sclerosis also known as Lou Gehrig's Disease	30,000 with 5,000 new cases yearly
ARTHRITIS	46.9 million diagnosed with it
ASTHMA	15.7 million people have it
BRONCHITIS	8.9 million with it
CANCER	16.0 million diagnosed
COPD Chronic Obstructive Pulmonary Disease	8.9 million
DIABETES	21 million Americans
HEART DISEASE	25.6 million diagnosed
HUNTINGTON'S DISEASE	30,000 known cases
KIDNEY DISEASE	3.8 million [42,762 deaths per year]
LIVER DISEASE	513,000 with 26,549 deaths per year
LUPUS	1.5 million
MULTIPLE SCLEROSIS	40,000 with MS with 200 diagnosed weekly
PARKINSON'S	1.5 million with 60,000 new cases yearly
STROKE	5.2 million per year

What's behind so much disease? I call it "The poisoning of America". It is by no accident that *more* than 1 out of every 2 people are "coming down" with such horrific diseases. In fact, in a different line of research I found that the "poisoning" of entire societies has happened in the past, and in my opinion is why many ancient societies simply vanished. Did you know that the Roman Empire (you know, the one that "fell") had decided to create their entire waterway structure (pipes) out of lead? It's undeniable, as archaelogists have unearthed huge chunks of their pipe, complete with Roman inscription. In addition, a photo on Wikipedia under "water pipe" shows an original Roman lead pipe with a folded seam at the Roman Baths in Bath, UK. Talk about mass poisoning! I believe firmly that we are experiencing a similar mass poisoning by the considerable amounts of mercury we are injecting into our bodies, placing permanently into teeth, and consuming in fish which are poisoned by our polluted waters.

Just *One* Of The Problems This is Causing

What follows is my "medical", "insurance", "IRS" story because it applies to many thousands if not millions of Americans. I have now suffered for a cumulative 44 years with the aforementioned health problems, all brought on by mercury. Our government has known about the dangers of mercury for centuries, but especially since 1930 as horror stories emerged about toxicities that were occuring with its use. The manufacturer of medical mercury (Eli Lily) was written many letters advising them to stop its use. This was all "swept under the rug". So here I am with major health issues that I wouldn't have if our government watchdogs had done their job. I've sought out doctors for help so many times that I now cannot get medical insurance.

Jump ahead now to 2008. I've taken every last penny out of my IRA fund to pay for therapies and aids in the hopes of reversing some of the disease. Of course we absolutely needed to alleviate some of the suffering as well. We spent over $90,000 in six years in the hopes of me not getting worse, so I can also help my husband not suffer so badly from his Parkinson's. What we are doing is effective in that we are both functioning and have minimal symptoms – so long as we can purchase and use the right organic foods, supplements, and natural therapies (simple therapies, like a massage chair for counteracting difficulty sleeping). But this all takes a lot of effort and time. One great therapy is making sure we get a good dose of sunshine (vitamin D3) daily. Between my own illnesses and my husbands, I went from being able to work full-time to only working a few hours here and there from home as time and strength would permit. I don't have insurance, so I pay for all aids and supplements for myself out of what I earn as I can. My husband's Medicare won't pay for "alternative" therapies and supplements, so we pay for those ourselves as well. We borrowed against our home to pay for it all. So what does the "government" *do* for us? Failed government policies have caused my suffering in the first place – and then they send me a letter telling me that they want over $10,000 in "penalties" for using my retirement money.

I relay this story because it just so happens that there are hundreds of thousands of people who are having very similar issues. Are you one of them? Politicians are campaigning that they will "fix" the healthcare crises. I want to challenge each reader of this book to write their own story as they begin to understand what really caused their suffering – and let's all "meet around the flagpole" in front of the White House one day and let our country know that in order to fix the healthcare crises you have to be correctly acknowledging the underlying cause. Our healthcare crises isn't because people don't have insurance (though everyone deserves insurance). Neither is our healthcare crises because medical costs are too high (although they *are* too high, but that's another story). **Our healthcare crises is because** *every other person* **is ill, their illness is severe requiring a lot of care –** *and they are severely ill because of pollutants.* "Insurance" doesn't work when only one of two people are paying for the insurance; the insurance policy is $300, $400 or $500 a month, and the "other" person is using up more than that for their healthcare!

So, not having insurance, I used my retirement money. I was told it was a sanctioned thing to do. My accountant xeroxed a page from an IRS guide book, entitled: Retirement Plans – Taxation of Benefits. It read:

2157 Penalty on Early Distributions. Generally, distributions from a qualified retirement plan are subject to an additional 10 percent penalty tax if they are made before the participant reaches age 59½. The 10 percent penalty tax will *not* apply to the portion of the early distribution that was timely and properly rolled over into an IRA or other qualified plan. *Exception to Penalty Tax.* Even when the distribution is not rolled over and is required to be included in the individual's gross income, the 10 percent penalty tax does *not* apply to:

Here they list many exceptions. Number 5 says:

(5) distributions not exceeding deductible medical expenses (determined without regard to whether deductions are itemized).

I was told by the tax man this means if you spent it all on medical (which we did), you don't pay the 10 percent penalty. That, of course, is entirely fair…especially considering I'm using up what was supposed to be my security for retirement (I only had about $35,000 left when this was taken out for medical expenses). Now I was using it for illnesses and suffering *caused* by the government failing to stop mercury in medicines and dentistry.

But then I received an email from my accountant which said that the IRS wanted a letter stating I'm disabled. My first reaction was to cry. I cogitated on the situation for a few days and then paid $2,500 to hire a lawfirm to put a freeze on my assets so the IRS can't just come in and take the tiny bit I have left. Again – I'm not alone.

To summarize:

I. Failed government watchdogs are allowing Americans to get sick in the first place, by allowing deadly substances like mercury be implanted into mouths and bodies. The diseases this one substance alone is causing, is the first and foremost reason for our "health and insurance crises".

2. Medical costs are rising through the roof so that those who can second-mortgage their house, or who have insurance will pay for those who do not.

3. People that do have insurance are using it for frequent and unnecessary trips to doctors, emergency rooms, testing, etc. I have witnessed this hundreds of times. Many are causing their own illnesses with smoking, drinking and extremely poor diet and lifestyle habits. Then there are unnecessary medical treatments. For example, my own husband partook of a couple of months of "speech therapy" just because they told him he could. The bill was thousands of dollars for that speech therapy. But we didn't pay for it – his "insurance" did. All he "learned" was that he needed to *speak louder.*

Now I don't write "complaints" without writing solutions… or at least suggested solutions.

They are:

1. It should be illegal to deny anyone insurance

2. All insurance cost should be based upon the income of the person…a percentage that is fair and affordable

3. Insurance should be like a savings account. It would work like this: You buy your insurance, and try hard not to use it, because a percentage of what you pay will come back to you, or roll-over into your "insurance savings" when you don't use it. This would make everyone want to only use their insurance for absolute necessities, not a sniffly nose because they don't take vitamin C or eat right. *Of course the "insurance" part is that you can never be denied any absolutely necessary medical care like heart bypass or kidney dialysis no matter how much it costs.*

4. We don't pay for the medical care of people who are in this country illegally especially if they aren't paying into the system.

Chapter 3
POLLUTANTS ARE KILLING US

Pollutants Are The Underlying Cause Of Disease

For most of my life I have been sick. I can't say that I remember ever waking up any day feeling wonderful. From age 11 on I've had psoriasis. As a pre-teen and teenager I've had more days with sore throats, eye sties, stomach aches, and herpes outbreaks than not. In my 20's when I was told I had lymphoma, I began twelve years of raw foods and various therapies, like drinking raw liver juice, wheatgrass juice and doing coffee enemas!

According to Dr. George T. Pack, MD, who was a cancer specialist at Cornell Medical School, almost everyone has cancer cells growing at all times. If the immune system is working properly, these cells are killed or reabsorbed by the defense system before they begin to grow and threaten health. The only real defense against cancer is the immune system. Cancer cells can multiply on any given day, but if the immune system is where it should be those cancer cells are eliminated and you are none the wiser. But if a person develops cancer severe enough to show up on tests, even though treatments may get it into remission, it can come back again unless the body conditions that allowed it to develop in the first place are corrected. Pollutants damage the immune system. *Pollutants* like mercury cause the cancer.

In my 30's began daily migraines, just feeling sick, always "recovering" from having yet another tooth worked on due to chronic decay or viral attacks on my nerves. In my 50's I began having the cramping, eyesight worsening, depression, clumsiness and misery of multiple sclerosis. When I was at a health resort years ago I encountered a gal who had overcome cancer (as I had after 12 years on a raw foods diet). She also did so by using raw foods and wheatgrass and such. When I asked her why she didn't shout it to the world, write a book, make the rounds with her story she said she was afraid that if she did, it would be like boasting, and the cancer would come back.

Indeed! Many, many people have overcome illnesses in their lifetimes. My mother tells the story of a young man she knew back during World War II days. He was told he had cancer and only a few months to live. They sent him home to die. He returned to his farm from the city where he'd been living. Then a miraculous thing happened - he got well – completely well. He didn't take the "King's medicines". He took God's. His was an "organic" farm (he was a small-time farmer...he didn't use pesticides like they do today). He lived out his complete lifespan.

It should come as no surprise whatsoever that pesticides contribute to and even cause neurological diseases. Most pesticides work by disabling the neurological system of pests! Most people know that pesticides are dangerous. I believe the problem lies in peoples' perception that by the time they consume a food, those pesticides have "disappeared". I believed similarly and *still* find it difficult to believe there are pesticide residues in any food I might eat. You can't taste them! But there most certainly are. Independent researchers have tested foods and found many fruits and vegetables to have pesticide residues, some more than others. In addition to pesticides, fruits and vegetables are also treated with other chemicals, like fungicides (which can contain mercury!)

Pesticides can cause **brain damage** and trigger conditions such as epilepsy, **multiple sclerosis** and **Parkinson's disease**, according to scientists. A landmark study claims that chemicals routinely used by farmers in the UK and around the world can result in **neurological diseases** [http://www.dailymail.co.uk/health/article-399684/Breathing-pesticides-trigger-MS-Parkinsons-disease.html]

Wanting to make sure that my husband and I weren't ingesting pesticides by eating two or three times per week at "Souplantation" (a huge salad bar restaurant found on the west coast), I sent a baggie of their salad to be tested at EMA labs in Woodland, California.

I also sent a baggie with an organic salad. The bags were labeled "A" and "B" so there would be no bias in the testing. Of the 159 mostly organophosphate types of pesticides for which they tested, the results came back that neither salad contained detectible pesticides. There was only one exception. The Souplantation salad had 0.02 ppm (tolerance level 1.0 ppm) of Chlorpyrifos (Dursban). The lab director told me this was barely detectible.

First I went to Souplantation and asked that they be brutally honest with me, and tell me how they handle their vegetables prior to serving. The manager launched into a pleasing tale of workers washing out the sink, sterilizing it, rinsing off vegetables, and then rinsing them again. Discussing this with EMA lab director David Elliott, I was told that certain pesticides are designed to go "systemically" into the plant, or stick so well to the plant *they cannot be washed off.* He also said that there are about 1,000 or so potential pesticides used worldwide (America does import food!) so having tested for 159 of the ones most commonly used in the U.S. cannot tell the entire story.

I wanted to be able to present my readers with some valuable information. I believe it is this:

1. Eat organic as much as you can — then you don't have to worry about whether there are pesticide residues or systemic pesticides, fungicides, herbicides.
2. Vitamin C is a natural and powerful detoxifier. Make sure you take it like a medicine daily. It is better to take 500 mg. at a time several times throughout each day than take high doses all at once, as it is a water-soluble vitamin and will be excreted within a couple of hours.
3. Don't live near farms that use pesticides. There is a city in California that grows lots of grapes. When I went there for a wedding I could smell chemicals in the air as if they lay like a sickening fog over the city. I'm sure the people who live there can no longer smell it. I'd love to know what their rate of cancer is.
4. Go online and search for "Pesticide Data Program" and find the United States Department of Agriculture's (usda.gov)

"Agricultural Marketing Service" Science and Technology program where they list how much pesticide has been found on various foods. Search until you find PDP Databases. There you will find year after year of reports you can download. Scroll down to the PDF reports and double click.

Some People Do Overcome Disease

It has been my experience that people who fight a disease like multiple sclerosis, even if they succeed in conquering it, or they figure out what caused it, are often in too much pain or too tired to share their findings. Or they feel like the gal at the health resort, and are afraid to share their success for fear of their disease returning. Indeed, after you've been beaten up by a disease you are often too tired to sit at a computer to revisit all the pain so you can document your journey. Perhaps you're disgusted and angry and don't believe anyone would believe your story, and thus benefit by your sharing anyway.

I've often said that if I could *really* pour out all I now understand about why every other person is getting migraines, lung cancer, MS, Parkinson's, Alzheimer's, etc., I would have to go out in the middle of the street and scream beyond my ability to scream, blood would pour out of every pore in my body, my brain would burst and I would die in the middle of the street from the weight of the truth. As I hear of yet another friend, relative or public figure getting cancer I feel like screaming. My sister-in-law has lung cancer, yet she's never smoked. Senator Ted Kennedy has brain cancer – and then I see him on the news after his diagnosis with a "Bluetooth" cell phone device in his ear (radiation!). Dana Reed died of lung cancer after her husband's battle with his paralysis, yet she was not a smoker. I want to scream when I hear of these people running to the doctor for *more* poisoning from chemo and radiation.

One day I realized that this must have been similar to Jesus taking the weight of all of our sins to the cross. He wasn't the only one to die on a cross, but He was the only one carrying the weight of all our sins! I'm not comparing myself to Jesus - just using Him as an analogy as to the *weight* of the burden of knowing truths others just can't seem to see. Unfortunately, the *true* cause of disease few really know: The mercury, the lead, the pesticides, the glutamates, the radiation, contributions of dentists, doctors and food manufacturers! If anyone is reading this who just doesn't get it, this isn't about being dramatic – if you *don't* get it, then it's because you haven't *yet* experienced the same degree of pain and misery as those of us afflicted with devastating diseases, and especially those of us who know why. We've been where you are, while you have yet to be where we are.

In fact, as a nutritionist, it occurred to me, because I pour over "scientific studies" for hours daily, writing papers, newsletters, brochures and more for doctors and healthcare professionals – that I could try to pull all of the studies together and *prove* to you "the cause of migraines" or "the cause of multiple sclerosis". Indeed, this book *is* pulling together studies, but the truth is, if we could "prove" the cause of any disease by merely pulling together studies, it would have been done long ago. People see studies and don't believe them! Or big business, with an interest to protect, pays to have "studies" done to disprove a study previously done! So you have to turn to God and Nature for the truth. When you have more than one out of every two people suffering, coupled with the fact that toxic metals, pesticides, and glutamates are freely used, combined with the fact that most people simply *don't* consume pure, whole foods on a daily basis – the truth should be obvious.

Because there are people or companies with money or reputations to lose by the truth coming out, the truth will be covered up (consider the Eli Lily case with thimerosal – next section). In addition, many truths have never been "scientifically" studied, because they don't make anyone any money! These truths are discredited. For example, why would someone spend the required multi-millions to *scientifically prove the efficacy of* an herb (that means double-blind, placebo-controlled trials, overseen by "authorities") that might even *cure* a disease, but couldn't then be sold for millions to make *back* the money spent, much less additional monies. The answer is, they won't, and they don't.

On the news today (December, 2008) came a story about an antioxidant that can prevent Alzheimer's. In this story the reporters kept showing a blue pill saying scientists combined high levels of B-vitamins with this "antioxidant". They blamed an elder person's inability to "create enough antioxidants" on the generation of Alzheimer's, and the neural damage seen in Alzheimer's on the lack of antioxidants. Studies actually show that *mercury* does the type of damage seen in Alzheimer's. If it were purely a lack of antioxidants, Alzheimer's would be far more rampant than it is, including in third world countries, and young people on the typical American junk food diet. We also know that getting old isn't synonymous with the inability to "create" anti-oxidants, but that a diet made up primarily of fresh, whole, raw fruits and vegetables is what supplies those antioxidants, and the precursors, along with other nutrients (like ample amino acids, minerals, etc.) for internally-produced antioxidants (like superoxide dismutase – a powerful antioxidant said to be deficient or "dysfunctional" in Alzheimer's). Older people are known for evolving to a diet made up of "comfort foods" like cookies, coffee, sandwiches, soups, etc. On the other hand, seniors are *not* known to consume copious quantities of pure, whole, raw, organic fruits and vegetables.

Studies have linked the antioxidant activity of melatonin, EGCG from green tea, and vitamin E to preventing the neural damage seen in Alzheimer's. In fact, the truth is actually hidden within thousands of studies that antioxidants in general protect us from *all* diseases. Un-fortunately older people are blindly trusting of their doctors, and say "yes" to that yearly flu shot with its thimerosal (mercury) without a second thought. While antioxidants are imperative – the fact remains, it is mercury that *causes* Alzheimer's.

Some People Seem To Do Everything Right, But...

My dental hygienist asked me how she could lose weight. During the course of telling her about the best foods for humans, and how eating them would naturally cause her to normalize her weight, she said she'd given up on natural foods because, "My mother was a com-plete health-foodist, and she died of cancer anyway".

I quizzed her as to her mother's diet, all the while knowing that *diet – good or bad, really, isn't what's killing us – pollutants are.* She told me about the many vegetables and fruits her mother ate. She told me of how her mother worked out regularly at the gym. She told me that her mother didn't have any "silver" fillings and wasn't accustomed to going to doctors. She was adamant that her mother was extraordinarily healthy. So when she got cancer and died at the age of 48, the girl confessed that she stopped believing you need to "eat healthy". I told her that *pollutants* are what are killing us, and that in order for her mother to have gotten cancer when she otherwise did everything right, she *had* to have been encountering a toxin source that led to her cancer. I asked if her mother ate fish. The girl said, *"every day — and often more than once a day."* Mercury.

Mercury Is Our Most Prevalent And Deadly Pollutant

In December, 2008, 43 year old actor, Jeremy Pivens was too sick and too weak to fulfill his contractual obligation, and left the cast of the Broadway revival of "Speed-the-Plow". We all saw it on the news. Reporters were saying that he just didn't want to do the play anymore, so he was faking being sick, saying he was "poisoned by mercury". But a month later Jeremy's doctor, Dr. Carlon Colker said that the actor was suffering from "extreme mercury toxicity". He went on to say that testing revealed that Jeremy had six times the "healthy" amount of mercury *(although there is no "healthy" amount — you're not supposed to have any mercury)*. So where did Mr. Pivens get all that mercury? He ate sushi, often twice a day. If Jeremy had been a "regular guy" (not "rich" or "famous") only his smaller circle of friends and family would ever have heard of his illness. And if true to form, these people would have dismissed his illness as either insignificant (he's merely tired), or from something else. And surely they would have thought him to be "crazy" for saying it was from mercury. In our society (although hopefully this will change with this book and more to follow) we're in total ignorance, disbelief and denial about what is causing our illnesses.

Thousands of tons of mercury are released into the air each year through pollution and waste. In the environment the mercury can transform into organic mercury, which is known as methylmercury, and accumulate in streams, oceans, water and soil. Methylmercury also accumulates in the food chain, so each fish absorbs the mercury in other fish and organisms it eats. For this reason, larger and older fish such as shark, tuna and swordfish contain the highest levels of methylmercury. [Dr. Joseph Mercola, www.mercola.com]

In fetuses and developing infants it can also have negative effects on attention span, language, visual-spatial skills, memory and coordination. It is estimated that nearly **60,000 children** each year are born at risk for **neurological problems** due to **methylmercury** exposure in the womb. [Dr. Joseph Mercola, www.mercola.com]

Mercury is in immunizations, dental materials, all products from the sea (from sea greens like spirulina and blue-green algae products to all fish) and more. And it's still in vaccines even though there is *proof* that Eli Lily (manufacturer of the mercury additive "thimerosal") in 1930, knew that it had devastating effects upon the immune and nervous system, and did everything to successfully (to this day) hide the truth! The Dallas-based law firm of Waters & Kraus announced in March 2002 that Eli Lilly's thimerosal product, the mercury-based vaccine preservative, has been implicated in a number of recent law suits as causing neurological injury to infants. Waters & Kraus emphasize that the danger of thimerosal has been known as early as April 1930. There is overwhelming proof that mercury has an affinity for the brain and central nervous system, and that it destroys the "battery" of your cells, the mitochondria, and thus *destroys* your immune system.

The World Health Organization (WHO) in 1991 listed the estimated average daily amount of mercury (in micrograms) that we're all taking in and being poisoned by. They also have emphatically declared that _no amount of mercury is safe._

SOURCE OF MERCURY	AVERAGE AMOUNT ABSORBED DAILY in mcg
Amalgam Fillings ["Silver" Fillings]	3.8 or more
Fish and Other Foods	3.0-3.6
Water	0.05
Air	0.04

Notice the World Health Organization doesn't even mention vaccines. It is unfathomable that they wouldn't know that thimerosal is mostly mercury and that a single hepatitis B shot can contain a whopping 12.5 mcg of the poison! Folks, to this day, thimerosal can *still* be in your flu vaccine and other vaccines. Thousands of parents are saying it caused their child's autism, and statistics show that about 1 in every 150 children born are getting autism, yet we *still* don't take it completely out of the vaccines.

"When I finished medical school **over 25 years ago**, the incidence of **autism was only one in 100,000**. Now it has conservatively climbed to 1 in 150, and some experts believe that if you consider the full range of neurological disorders that could logically be under the umbrella "Autism Spectrum Disorder" the incidence may be as high as one in 10." http://rss.mercola.com/NL/rss.aspx

One in ten! My nephew got epilepsy after a series of vaccinations. I remember him standing on his little stepstool to brush his teeth at about two years of age. He'd had a vaccination very recently. His little lip quivered uncontrollably. Neurological damage. He went on to develop full-blown epilepsy, and battles it to this day as an adult. The damage from the mercury in those immunizations has definitely made his life include far more suffering, work and expense than there should have been.

So its not just autism. Mercury damage to the brain/neurological system would result in any of a number of conditions including attention deficit disorder, Tourette's syndrome, autism, epilepsy and depression to name a few.

In early 2008 the parents of 9-year-old Hannah who had autism, won a lawsuit and federal compensation because of their child's autism being caused by the mercury in her vaccines. Hannah's father, Dr. Jon Poling, a neurologist in private practice in Athens, Georgia (Hannah's mother is a lawyer) paved the way for others seeking the same recognition and compensation. But is that what it takes? Do you have to be a doctor, a lawyer, or have money to have the truth validated? [Note: As of October 2008, a total of 12,746 lawsuits have been filed with claims that the mercury in immunization caused the child's autism. Of these 2,266 have been compensated while 4,755 have been dismissed.]

Infant primates given vaccines on U.S. children's immunization schedule develop behavioral symptoms of **autism**. Http://www.detoxmetals.com/vaccines-and-autism.html

In addition our military are being injected with mercury at extraordinarily high rates. This fact correlates with a high incidence of Lou Gehrig's (a neurological disorder of the worst kind) among the military. If you've ever met someone with Lou Gehrig's you know it's something *nobody* deserves. It has also come out that you have many times more chance of getting Alzheimer's (another neurological disease) if you've had regular flu shots (mercury).

Hugh Fudenberg, MD, an immunogeneticist with nearly 850 papers published in peer review journals, has reported that if an individual had five consecutive **flu shots** between 1970 and 1980 (the years studied), his/her **chances of getting Alzheimer's Disease** is **ten times higher** than if they had less shots. From the Univ of Kentucky, Dr. Boyd Haley has done extensive research in the area of mercury toxicity and the brain, in collaboration with researchers at University of Calgary. Haley stated that "seven of the characteristic markers that we look for to distinguish Alzheimer's disease can be produced in normal brain tissues, or cultures of neurons, by the addition of extremely low levels of mercury." [Dr Sherri Tenpenny www.nmaseminars.com 11-30-03]

The scientific proof *is* freely available, for example, there are hundreds of thousands of studies available at www.pubmed.gov, but most people will never see them. Others wouldn't understand the vernacular even if they did see them. Like the quote below. The important thing it is saying is that one thing mercury does is lead to inflammation, a dangerous and painful component of so many diseases.

> **Mercury** causes release of **inflammatory cytokines** such as Tumor Necrosis Factor-alpha (TNFa) and Interleukin-4 which are documented to be factors in the chronic inflammatory conditions discussed here, including asthma, lupus, rheumatoid arthritis, scleroderma, celiac and Crohn's disease, etc. and also is involved in chronic heart problems. [Bernard Windham(Ed.)

Many who see the truth in writing, even if they understand it, won't often believe it. (Remind you of anything? How about the people who saw Jesus' miracles, and *still* didn't believe!) I believe the bewilderment, astonishment, and confusion is because we just *can't* believe that our benevolent dentists and doctors and government would *allow* mercury to be used in the way it is. But our government is made up of imperfect humans, and they *do* allow it. Partially they don't know or understand, and partially they put their head down in the sand because it's easier than dealing with the truth, as well as any loss of income!

Mercury Destroys Your Protective Systems

Mercury, and other toxic metals (like **cadmium** from cigarette smoke) have a high affinity for sulfhydryl (-SH) groups, thus inactivating numerous enzymatic reactions, amino acids, and sulfur-containing antioxidants such as N-acetylcysteine (NAC), alpha lipoic acid (ALA) and glutathione (GSH). These antioxidants are the body's premier defense *against* mercury and other toxic metals and substances. Mercury (also cadmium, and likely other toxic metals) *wipes them out*. Without the protection afforded by these antioxidants, bodywide damage ensues. Mercury and cadmium both bind to metallothionein. Mercury, because toxic metals substitute for beneficial trace metals like zinc, reduces the effectiveness of metalloenzymes. This is spelled out in the publication *The role of mercury and cadmium heavy metals in vascular disease, hypertension, coronary heart disease, and myocardial infarction.* By MC Houston. Published in *Ther Health Med*, Vol 13, No 2 (2007)

Intracellular GSH status appears to be a sensitive indicator of the cells overall health, and its ability to resist toxic challenges. According to **Dr. Boyd Haley** of the University of Kentucky..."**Autism...is ALL about the glutathione**" http://www.y2khealthanddetox.com/gshcomplex.html

In the above box, Dr. Haley states that autism is "all about glutathione". Glutathione is a detoxifying compound made within the body and is used up by nearly every toxic assault upon the body, including mercury (more about glutathione in the next section). Study after study shows many people with various diseases are "low in glutathione". All three of the main diseases covered in this book, psoriasis, migraines and multiple sclerosis have studies showing that people suffering from these diseases are low in glutathione. Why? Because the toxic material (mercury) that caused the disease used up this detoxifying compound. If the toxic assault is far greater than the body's ability to manufacture glutathione, the toxic compound wins. So the truth is, autism is all about *mercury* and mercury depletes glutathione.

As immunizations rose from a single shot for smallpox to over 50 shots within the first couple years of life – and all that mercury – the incidence of autism rose from less than one in 2,000 to one in every 150 children. When only one in 2,000 used to get autism they would have done so from other mercury use, like heavy consumption of seafood, or amalgams placed or topical applications (it was used in medications like mercurochrome for example).

You Can't Treat The Disease Unless You Know What Caused It

The danger of not knowing the absolute truth lies in how you go about treating the disease and its symptoms. When you don't know the true underlying cause, and you attempt to treat one of the many "things going on", you can easily mistreat and do more harm than good. For example, with diseases that involve damage to the glutama-tergic system by mercury, *giving glutathione* in the form of an injection or supplements can do further damage. Glutathione is made up of the amino acids glycine, cysteine and glutamine! In someone with a dam-aged glutamatergic system, instead of glutathione behaving like the antioxidant it is, it will more likely break down into its three amino acids and supply more excitotoxic glutamine to an already damaged brain and central nervous system.

Mercury *causes* a loss of glutathione. Scientists and doctors alike know very well that glutathione is one of the body's master detoxifi-ers. If you are rushed to the hospital with an acetaminophen overdose (Tylenol) and the emergency room doctors *know* what's wrong with you (therein lies the rub) you'll be given NAC, which contains cyste-ine, a sulfur-containing amino acid, and one of the building blocks of glutathione, in the hopes of saving your life against the toxic effects of the Tylenol.

Plants also need protection against toxins. Plants are made up of cells, just like humans and these cells have similar challenges to our own cells. Isn't this interesting:

A **zinc deficiency** has been induced in *Coffea arabica* trees in Kenya Colony as a result of spraying with fungicidal formulations contain-ing **mercury** in organic combination. The symptoms were first ob-served in October 1957 on coffee trees which had been treated with certain mercurial sprays against coffee berry disease (*Colletotrichum coffeanum* Noack). [*Nature* 182, 1607 - 1608 (06 December 1958); doi:10.1038/1821607a0]

For quite some time I wanted to find out just where mercury would sit on a list of the earth's most toxic substances. Then in Au-gust, 2008, I stumbled onto the government's "Center For Disease Control" list of over 250 toxic substances, and where they rank in toxicity. See below. Note that plutonium, radon and uranium aren't listed likely where they should be, at number 1, 2 or 3 and I'm guessing that is because those three highly toxic substances simply aren't normally found in the average American's daily life.

2007 RANK	SUBSTANCE NAME	TOTAL POINTS	2005 RANK	CAS #
1	ARSENIC	1672.58	1	007440-38-2
2	LEAD	1534.07	2	007439-92-1
3	MERCURY	1504.69	3	007439-97-6

This is from a chart of over 250 toxic substances listed in order of toxicity. Note that mercury is #3. A dentist puts it in your mouth? Doctors are injecting it directly into your body? Found at: http://www.atsdr.cdc.gov/cercla/07list.html

I would find it humorous if it weren't so tragic that we are still being told to eat fish, that its good for us, but to just choose fish with less mercury. *There is no safe level of mercury.* If you are being told to eat fish by any "agency", it is because the fish industry is paying to have you told to eat fish.

Pay no attention to those who say "there is only a *trace*" of mercury. Mercury is cumulative, meaning as you consume more it adds to what you've already consumed, *building up* in toxicity. Toxic metals accumulate in tissue, like in bone marrow. But before it settles anywhere (some leaves the body via detox routes) it does damage as shown graphically in a powerful film out of the University of Calgary, Canada. (See Chapter 9 *Multiple Sclerosis*)

There is a chart found at http://tuberose.com/Graphics/fish-poster.jpg (you can also right click and save it to your own computer) telling you how to pick fish lower in mercury. I don't use this chart to choose fish lower in mercury, because I don't want *any* mercury! I *do* use this chart to prove that *all* fish is tainted with mercury, and you can do the same.

Besides Mercury, Another Pollutant We Cannot Ignore Is Lead

Lead is a highly toxic metal and has been a problem for many years. Many of our cities (if not all) currently use lead solderings to join water pipes and thus lead can be found in tap water. Everyone needs to use a multi-system water purification system before consuming their faucet water. There are also showerhead purifiers that can be purchased for bathing.

But lead is also currently being found in products from China. When I began writing this section in May of 2008, I predicted that, if it doesn't get covered up, it won't be long, and we'll find that *all* products from China have major contaminants. So far it's going in that direction. We've now seen toys, drywall, dental crowns, heparin, jewelry, zorries and electronic equipment tainted with toxic substances (so far, mostly lead, but also melamine as I discuss later).

Then in December, 2008 a television news magazine showed the testing of many products from China, using a lead testing "gun". *Everything* that was tested contained lead to varying degrees. I was stunned to watch as a little canvas purse contained lead! I searched for a similar "gun" to see if it was affordable for the average person to own. I found that a similar device is called the X-MET 3000 TXR+ available at www.metorex.com (800) 229-9209 (Oxford Instruments). The "gun" is made in Finland, but sold through a distributor in New Jersey. They say that the lead scanner will test products for not only lead but also arsenic, cadmium, mercury, chrome, nickel and other hazardous metals. Unfortunately, however, this instrument is not affordable for the average person.

Children Being Poisoned By Lead

On a recent episode of the television show, "Extreme Home Makeover" a family with neurologically ill foster children were having their home redone. Ken and Doreen Silva had helped over a dozen foster children over the years but they were told to cease and desist because the kids have all tested positive for lead poisoning. This family was lucky to have their home redone, but even more lucky that their neurologically-challenged children were tested at their school for heavy metal poisoning, and high levels of lead were found. This led to the testing of their soil and home surroundings and this is where lead contamination was discovered. When I watched this I thought to myself (after China came to mind) that this family was fortunate to have school officials take it upon themselves to test their children. I propose that there are hundreds of thousands if not millions of children and homes that would yield similar test results but either no-one thinks to do the testing, no-one knows how to get testing done, or the testing is financially out of reach for the average family. Sad.

Why Is China Putting Lead Into "Everything"?

Last year I saw a documentary showing little Chinese kids sitting around a fire. They were burning old computer monitors sent to them by the U.S.A. Are they now sending us back our poisons? Actually *I wouldn't blame them if they are!* How *dare* we send such toxic materials to them in the first place!

In 2002, the Basel Action Network was co-author of a report that said 50 percent to 80 percent of **electronics waste collected for recycling** in the United States was being disassembled and recycled under largely unregulated, unhealthy conditions in **China**, India, Pakistan and other developing countries. The new report contends that Americans may be lulled into thinking their old computers are being put to good use. [See story and devastating photo at: http://www.nytimes.com/2005/10/24/technology/24junk.html or look up: "Poor Nations Are Littered With Old PCs" by Laurie J. Flynn, 2005]

Computer monitors (the cathode ray tube kind) have about 5 pounds of lead in each one:

It turns out that the **glass in a CRT contains a lot of lead**. A big CRT can contain up to **5 pounds (2.2 kilograms) of lead**. [http://computer.howstuffworks.com/question678.htm]

I wonder if the Chinese discovered we were sending this devastating neurological toxin to their country by the tons, got angry, and decided to quietly repackage it and ship it right back to us? It's in *everything.* I previously mentioned two young children who died from swallowing little jewelry trinkets from China that contained lead. But again, toxins are turning up in *so many things* – for example there were photos on the internet of zorries from China causing major blistering and inflammation of the feet of the wearer.

An emailed message included several photographs depicting a woman's feet with **a severe skin reaction** apparently caused by **a pair of rubber flip flops** (usually called "thongs" in Australia and "jandals" in New Zealand). The message claims that chemicals used in the manufacture of the flip flops caused the rash. According to the message, the flip flops were **made in China** and sold cheaply in Wal-Mart stores in the US. The case described in the message is **true** and the photographs are genuine. [http://www.hoax-slayer.com/flip-flops-china-rash.shtml]

Lou Dobbs

A report on December 6th, 2008 airing of Lou Dobbs was entitled, "Toxic Toys – Dangerous Toys Still On Shelves". The question posed was *why*? Why are there still toxic toys on the shelf!? These toys came from China. February 10th, 2009 is the date that toxic toys can no longer be *manufactured*...but they can still be sold after that date!! Go to www.healthytoys.org to get a list of those tested. These toys contain lead, mercury, formaldehyde and more.

My greatest respect and love goes out to Lou Dobbs. He raged after this report, and asked his staff *who is on that committee allowing this?* How can they sleep at night? He said "I want their names!" He "invited" them (said, 'if they've got the guts') he wants them to come and answer to this outrage of allowing toxic toys to still be sold to America's children.

If you don't think it's outrageous, imagine, if you will, the most precious little person in your life swallowing a little trinket made in China. You didn't know they swallowed it – much less know what they swallowed was made in China. Suddenly they get very ill and die. It's not until an autopsy is done that they find that trinket lodged in their gut somewhere. I picture my precious granddaughter – and I'm outraged.

The Truth About Toxic Imports From China Has Been All But Shelved

I'd like to say that this has all been "front page news"...but it really hasn't been, including a story just in March, 2008, of dental crowns from China filled with lead.

Dentists who use cut-price and potentially deadly **crowns and dentures from China** are putting their patients at risk, it was claimed today. The products are often made in unregulated laboratories and can contain **dangerous levels of lead**, dental experts warned. In the U.S., four cases of lead poisoning have been linked to Chinese dental fixtures. A laboratory test revealed that some contained **210 times the acceptable amount** of the toxic metal. [http://www.dailymail.co.uk/news/article-528615/Cheap-dental-crowns-China-contain-dangerous-levels-LEAD.html#]

Did you get that? 210 times the acceptable amount! Understand, however, that with arsenic, mercury and lead, there is really <u>no</u> *acceptable* amount. Unfortunately, at this point in time, I believe you can't trust *anything* from China. I now refuse to purchase anything from China, and yet it still sneaks into my house - like a Macintosh monitor that says "assembled in China". Until this issue is resolved, I go out of my way to put back anything I buy, or throw away anything I bought previously that was made in China. I let a store clerk know – "oops, sorry – I have to put that back, it was made in China – we boycott their products until proven to not contain any toxic materials". Of course, this is nearly impossible shopping in Wal-Mart, Lowe's or other "discount" type stores - so I rarely shop there anymore. I had an armful of games once in Toys R Us, ready to buy, and then noticed every single one was made in China. I went back to the shelves and found only two USA manufacturers of the 30 or so game makers! The USA games cost twice what the ones made in China cost, but I gladly paid the price.

<u>May, 2008 the headlines say</u>:

Greenpeace: Game Consoles Contain Dangerous Chemical Levels. They're talking about "Nintendo Co. Ltd.'s (NTDOY) Wii, the Sony Corp. (SNE) Playstation 3 and Microsoft Corp.'s (MSFT) Xbox 360 use varying degrees of bromine, PVCs and other potentially harmful chemicals, including phthalates which can affect human hormones." The news release tells us we're in no "immediate danger". I beg to differ. But trying to keep the public in the dark about the danger is a good example of how officials attempt to keep people from panicking. The goal is to keep us from taking back products we've purchased or refusing to buy products, thus affecting the economy. Little of what you're told is the absolute truth, nor with the proper concern not only for your personal health, but the health of the world as a whole. The *truth* is, the toxic chemicals that these products contain (and I predict we'll learn over the next 10 years or sooner that most *everything* man-made contains dangerous chemicals) *do* pose immediate concern as molecules of the chemicals waft up into air, are thrown into our landfills, get into our water, rub off on our skin and more. Remember: *One out of every two people are coming "down" with a devastating disease — and, no, it's <u>not</u> because you're stressed, don't exercise, or because you eat red meat. And yes, it <u>is</u>* from highly toxic chemicals completely and often irreversibly disrupting the normal functioning of your 10-100 trillion body cells. Now, *please* tell me you're at least *beginning* to understand.

<u>Another headline reads</u>:

March. 5, 2008 WASHINGTON - Baxter International Inc. has found signs of a possible **contaminant in the recalled blood thinner heparin** that caused hundreds of serious side effects in the United States, which further points suspicion at ingredient suppliers in **China**.

<u>An October, 2008 headline reads</u>:

"The Melamine-tainted trail" and was published in The Los Angeles Times. It tells of eggs, biscuits, chocolate, cookies, and candy that were tainted with a toxic substance melamine (used in the production of plastics and destroys the kidneys), that all come from, you guessed it, China. Melamine-laced formula killed four babies and sickened more than 50,000. It was used to boost protein readings in the products! But it was also used in the feed given to chickens and even put into pesticides. So this article (as do I) recommends that anything from China best be considered suspect until proven safe. I'll add here that purchasing only pure, fresh, whole, (preferably organic) foods grown locally is another way to ensure safety. If you don't buy foods with an "ingredient list" (meaning they are fresh and whole, not "man-made") you're just that much further ahead on the safety scale.

Nickel Is Carcinogenic, Is It In Your Mouth?

Your mouth should be metal free. "Pure gold" would be okay, but its too soft, so they must add other metals to it. One common addition is nickel. Nickel is highly toxic.

> **Nickel** is a known hematotoxic, immunotoxic, hepatotoxic, pulmo-toxic, and nephrotoxic agent. [Das KK et al. Effect of nickel exposure on peripheral tissues: role of oxidative stress in toxicity and possible protection by ascorbic acid. *Rev Environ Health.* 2007 Apr-Jun;22(2):157-73.]

Every gold crown in my own mouth rotted underneath, and I suspect nickel is the reason. Most people likely have rotting underneath their crowns and don't even know it. The study above is saying that nickel is toxic to the blood, the immune system, the liver, the lungs and the kidneys. It just doesn't get any worse. Nickel is a known carcinogenic. So you're okay with it under your crowns with a "direct line" to your bloodstream?

Nitrites Create Nitric Oxide Which Precurses a Migraine

Nitrites are found in many processed foods, especially processed meats like bacon, lunch meats and sausages. Nitrites create nitric oxide, the precursor to migraines and other inflammatory conditions (see Chapter 8 *Migraines*). This is why the ideal diet for every human being would be made up of pure, fresh, whole, (preferably organic) foods, as they would be devoid of toxic food additives. Perhaps the most toxic food additive is monosodium glutamate (see below), and like mercury, is in the "worst" category because of its *prevalence* as well as its toxicity. Of course there are many other chemicals added to our foods that are also very damaging, like nitrites. Yet once your body is damaged and you go to the doctor seeking help, unfortunately, *never* does your doctor say, "Do you consume free glutamates or nitrites?" Why? He most certainly should investigate the possible toxins affecting your health!

Neither does your doctor recommend that you make *sure* you take in copious amounts of antioxidants every single day to stand guard at your cells against toxic chemicals. If doctors were completely honest, they would tell their patients they can't help them unless they stop smoking, drinking excessively, eating foods laden with toxic chemicals, etc. They don't say this for three reasons. One is that they'd be hippocrits (engaging in many of these things themselves); secondly they would lose all their patients because they'd get well; and third is because they simply don't *know* enough about the true cause of disease.

Cured meats are high in **nitrites**. Nitrites generate reactive nitrogen species that may cause damage to the lung. The objective is to assess the relation between frequent consumption of cured meats and the risk of newly diagnosed **chronic obstructive pulmonary disease** (COPD). [Varraso R et al. Prospective study of cured meats consumption and risk of chronic obstructive pulmonary disease in men. *Am J Epidemiol.* 2007 Dec 15;166(12):1438-45.]

Nitrites "reduce" to nitric oxide in the body. *Nitric oxide* is the molecule that directly precurses a migraine, an asthma attack, and many other maladies.

Significantly **higher nitrite concentrations** were found in **migraine** patients, with and without aura, and cluster headache patients, in remission and cluster phase, than in controls. These findings suggest that a basal dysfunction in the L-arginine-NO pathway may be involved in the peripheral mechanisms predisposing subjects with neurovascular headaches to individual attacks. [*Cephalgia* 2002 Feb;22(1):33-6]

If you take a sample of urine of migraineurs during a migraine attack, you'll find that their nitric oxide levels are significantly higher than on non-migraine days, and than in people who do not get migraines.

This study evaluated a relationship between **nitric oxide (NO) and migraine** attacks in order to gain insight into migraine pathomechanism. All subjects collected morning urine samples for 40 consecutive days. Urinary NO metabolites, nitrite/nitrate (NO(x)) levels were measured… mean urinary NO(x)/Cr ratio and number of NO(x) **peaks was significantly greater in the migraine group. NO(x) peaks coincided with headache days.** [Goadsby P et al. Increased urinary excretion of nitric oxide metabolites in longitudinally monitored migraine patients. *Eur J Neurol.* 2006 Dec;13(12):1346-51.]

There are many precursors to the body's own production of nitric oxide, and these are discussed more thoroughly in Chapter 8 *Migraines.*

Phthalates Are In Plastics

There's an email circulating that goes like this:
WARN YOUR MOTHERS/WIVES/GIRLFRIENDS AND DAUGHTERS
Bottled water in your car.....can be very dangerous to women!!!! This is how Sheryl Crow got breast cancer. In fact Sheryl was on the Ellen show and said this same exact thing. This has been identified as the most common cause of the high levels in breast cancer, especially in Australia. A friend, whose mother was recently diagnosed with breast cancer, the doctor told her:

Women should not drink bottled water that has been left in a car. The doctor said that the heat and the plastic of the bottle have certain chemicals that can lead to breast cancer. So please be careful and do not drink bottled water that has been left in a car, and, pass this on to all the women in your life. This information is the kind we need to know and be aware and just might save us!!!! The heat causes toxins from the plastic to leak into the water and they have found these toxins in breast tissue. Use a stainless steel Canteen or a glass bottle when you can!!! Let every one that has a wife/girlfriend and daughter know please.

It's true, there are "chemicals" (see below) in plastic that are carcinogenic (in the case of plastics these chemicals are "endocrine" (hormone) disrupters) and don't belong in your body. But what is left out here is that these chemicals are dangerous to men, women, children, dogs, cats – *all living creatures* – probably even plants! Also left out is the fact that its not just by leaving the bottle in your car that is dangerous. In fact, that may even be the least of your worries, because warm water left in the car is usually discarded because the water takes on a plastic taste – most people throw it away and start with a new bottle.

Here's a personal story. I heard about the plastic issue about 3 or 4 years ago. Up to that time we'd been avid plastic water bottle purchasers and drinkers. It was not uncommon for us to buy 3 or 4 cases at a time at Costco every month. Then one day I was pulling into a "mini mart" type of gas station, and noticed a flat of water bottles piled about 10 cases high out in the hot sun. It occurred to me then, that even if I didn't keep my water bottle in the heat, the store may have gotten the bottles from a hot warehouse, a hot truck, or even left them out in the hot sun. I couldn't win. Plastic had to go.

Of course its not just plastic water bottles. You shouldn't cook in a microwave with plastic wrap around or over your food either. Actually, we don't cook in a microwave at all because by virute of it cooking with unnatural "micro waves", we know it can chemically alter the natural structure of food. It was difficult, but we began warming up our soup in a stainless steel or glass soup pan (no aluminum, no Teflon). Yes, we have to wash two things now, not just the bowl. But we've quickly adjusted.

Basically, you need to "go green" in everything you do and everything you consume. Begin to learn one day at a time what is "natural", and what contains dangerous chemicals.

Humans have significant exposures to **phthalates,** as these chemical plasticizers are ubiquitously present in flexible plastics. Recent epidemiological evidence indicates that boys born to women exposed to phthalates during pregnancy have an increased incidence of **congenital genital malformations and spermatogenic dysfunction,** signs of a condition referred to as testicular dysgenesis syndrome (TDS). [*Reprod Toxicol.* 2007 Apr-May;23(3):366-73.]

Phthalates Mutate Your Brain's Neurons

In Chapter 9 – *Multiple Sclerosis* you'll learn that your brain's neurons are made up of two proteins:

Brain neurons have central cell bodies and processes. At the end of each neurite are growth cones where structural proteins are assembled to form the cell membrane. Two principal proteins involved are **actin** (responsible for the pulsating motion in neurons) and **tubulin.** Tubulin molecules link together to form the neurite membrane.

Studies show that phthalates interefere with the protein actin, which is responsible for the motility of your neurons (their ability to "pulsate" or move). Phthalates *mutate* actin and thus your neurons. All to say that phthalates are yet another pollutant that we need to avoid as we increase our awareness that *pollutants* are first and foremost what are *causing* the world's epidemic of diseases.

We previously reported that transient administration of **phthalates** induced **actin** cytoskeleton disruption... Results indicated a modification of actin distribution after phthalate administration. The present study also supports the **mitogenic effects of phthalates**... benzyl butyl phthalate treated cells, suggested a possible effect of the **endocrine disruptor in cancer processes**. [*J Cell Biochem.* 2007 Jun 1;101(3):543-51.]

Not surprisingly, a government website says that they have found no connection between phthalates and cancer. Typical denial so as not to alarm or cause an epidemic of lawsuits.

Studies show that **phthalates are "endocrine disruptors"**. This means your normal hormones are mutated, waylaid, disrupted, stopped, increased excessively, etc. Your hormones are your body's master orchestrators. When they are "disrupted" *anything* can happen, such as cancer. It has been known for decades that excessive estrogen, for example, leads to excessive cell growth – cancer.

The **phthalates** are ubiquitous industrial plasticizers and include agents such as di(2-ethylhexyl) phthalate (DEHP), dibutyl phthalate (DBP), and butyl benzyl phthalate (BBP), which are classified as **endocrine disruptors** because of their anti-androgenic or **pro-estrogenic effects**. [*J Toxicol Environ Health A.*2005 Dec 10;68(23-24):1995-2003.]

The fact that phthalates are ubiquitous (meaning they are *everywhere*) and that they are "anti-androgenic" (androgenic - pertaining to the development of male characteristics) is something to ponder as well. How is it, I often wonder, that a man can be born a man, but doesn't *feel* like a man? How is it, indeed, that we have *millions* of men who prefer men and women who prefer women? Of *course* God designed that men prefer women and women prefer men as proven by how God created men and women to reproduce. I love all people, and have no criticism whatsoever for *anyone.* In fact, as a "scientist" of sorts, I believe all people feel what they feel because of what's going on physically inside their bodies. I refer to the above study.

That said, there are many chemicals that can function as "endocrine disruptors", not just plastics.

An endocrine disruptor (ED) is, therefore, defined as a foreign substance or mixture that alters function(s) of the endocrine system, consequently harming an individual life form, its offspring, or population. [www.greenfacts.org]

We know that since earliest recorded history man has been harnassing and compounding dangerous chemicals, even mercury, lead and arsenic – all of which are highly toxic to the body, any of which could disrupt normal hormonal function. But even "unrecorded" history proves this to be true, as containers of dangerous chemicals have been found in tombs and in archaeological digs.

Mercury occurs naturally in the environment as mercuric sulfide, also known as cinnabar. It is also present in some fossil fuels. Cinnabar has been refined for its mercury content since the 15th or 16th century B.C. Its health hazards have been known at least since the Roman conquest of Spain. Due to the toxicity of mercury in cinnabar, criminals sentenced to work in quicksilver mines by the Romans had a life expectancy of only 3 years. [http://www.ingham.org/HD/LEPC/pamphlets/hazwaste/mercuryfacts.html]

A 2006 study documents the finding of toxic lead sediment in the "Egyptian Old Kingdom" which for them proved civilization in the area from 2686-2181 B.C. and then another layer with lead from 1000-800 B.C. For me, it proves man has been harnassing highly toxic substances for thousands of years, and has been suffering the consequences for the same period of time. [Veron A et al. Pollutant lead reveals the pre-Hellenistic occupation and ancient growth of Alexandria, Egypt. *Geophysical research letters.* 2006, vol. 33, no 6].

By 650 B.C. the list of chemicals may be said to include Common Salt, *Sal gemma*, red *Sal Gemma*, Lime, Saltpeter from the earth, Carbonate of Soda from the walls, Nitrate of Potash from walls, Sal Ammoniac [used in the Lalande Cell], Alkali from plants, Gypsum, Mercury from cinnabar, Alum, Black and Yellow Sulphur, Bitumen, various forms of Arsenic, red and black Copper Oxide, Chrysocolla, Haematite, Magnetic Iron Ore, Iron Pyrites (which leads to Vitriols), Iron Sulphide, Copper Sulphate; and if I am right, they had a word *hannabahru* for the fuming sulphuric acid from Green Vitriol. [*A Survey of the Chemistry of Assyria in the Seventh Century B.C.*, from AMBIX, Vol. II, No. I, June 1938]

Headline: Bisphenol-A (BPA) In Plastics Harming Humans

CNN ran a story: "Failing FDA: New Evidence BPA Poses Risks" September, 2008. The story told how the FDA continues to maintain that BPA is safe, but scientists have detected 93% of BPA in humans *causing neural and behavioral effects* at the current exposure levels. Canada has declared BPA a hazardous material. So why is BPA still allowed in baby bottles, plastic bottles, linings in cans, and more? I think the cat was out of the bag when the FDA alluded to how "important" the chemical is in these products.

BPA is a chemical used to make polycarbonate plastic and epoxy resins. Polycarbonate plastic is a lightweight and high-performance plastic. It is known for its strength and glass-like appearance. It is used in CDs, DVDs, electrical and electronic equipment, the automobile industry, and food and drink containers. It is a toxic substance when ingested, so the main concern with BPA is that which is used in food containers, like the protective liners in metal cans as well as baby bottles.

Folks, it's the same story repeated over and over. We use highly toxic chemicals as long as the "benefit" appears to outweigh the risk. It isn't until hundreds of thousands fall horribly ill to these chemicals (if, indeed, they are ever told the truth as to what caused their illness) that we even begin to think there is any reason to place health above convenience (in this case using glass instead of plastic).

Pesticides Are Neurotoxic

You would never expect your dog to remain healthy if you put a "drop" of pesticides in his water daily! Yet that is what you're getting (or *more*) by consuming commercially-grown foods. Most pesticides do the job of killing pests by destroying their neurological system. Others do the job by disrupting some aspect of an insect's life cycle. My question is, what aspect of *your* life cycle will the ingestion of that pesticide disrupt? I can't believe man thinks *nothing* will happen to him when he ingests pesticides!

There are environmental conditions and contaminates that can cause common neurological symptoms of numbness, tingling, paresthesia, pain, and weakness. Would you recognize the symptoms of **neurotoxicity**? Only the astute doctor of chiropractic is going to evaluate the possibility of lead toxicity, arsenic poisoning, solvent or **pesticide exposure**. Increasing use of chemicals in our workplaces and home environments suggests that all clinicians should be aware of potential overlap into their specialty. [By David P. Gilkey, DC, MEPM http://www.chiroweb.com/mpacms/dc/article.php?id=38255]

Look for organic! All commercially grown foods are most likely tainted with pesticides. Based on over 100,000 recent U.S. Government tests, on 46 popular fruits and vegetables, The Environmental Working Group (EWG), a non profit consumer watchdog group, came up with the "Dirty Dozen." This is a grouping of 12 commercially grown fruits and vegetables that have the highest levels of toxic pesticide residue. Even with this list, however, it is still best to strive to purchase everything organic. I spoke with a lab director who told me that if there are pesticide residues on your fruits or vegetables, they are there because they've been designed to cling to the food. *They cannot be washed off.* He told me has to laugh at all the soaps and washes designed to wash off these residues. "They don't work", he said.

The "Dirty Dozen":

1. Strawberries
2. Bell peppers (green and red)
3. Spinach (tied with number 2)
4. Cherries (grown in the United States)
5. Peaches (grown in Chile)
6. Cantaloupe (grown in Mexico)
7. Celery
8. Apples
9. Apricots
10. Green beans
11. Grapes
12. Cucumbers

Persistent Organic Pollutants

Throughout history man has used very toxic substances that took many obvious illnesses or deaths before the realization of danger occured. One is **DDT** (Dichloro-diphenyl-trichloroethane) a potent insecticide now only used for the prevention of malaria in specific regions of the world. DDT is very toxic, very persistent in the environment, and is hence classified as a "persistent organic pollutant" or POP. Another POP is PCB. PolyChlorinated Biphenyls are a mixture of up to 209 chlorinated chemicals that are also highly toxic, and thankfully no longer produced in the United States.

Unfortunately, just as the name implies, "persistent organic pollutants" can persist for many decades in the fatty tissue of the human body and in the environment. One very recent (2008) study out of Korea discusses the results of several epidemiological studies linking a substance in the human body called serum gamma-glutamyltransferase (GGT) to diabetes. GGT is an enzyme that is necessary for amino acids to join and form a peptide (a protein). The Korean study noted that GGT activity was related to diabetes in that its activity was found during the body's production of glutathione. Glutathione happens to be a "tripeptide" made up of the amino acids glutamic acid, cysteine and glycine.

Recall that GGT is needed to assemble these amino acids. Glutathione is perhaps the body's most important and powerful detoxifier. Glutathione protects the liver, the kidneys, indeed, all your cells from toxic substances. In fact, every time you take aceteminophen (Tylenol) your body uses glutathione to detoxify your liver of the drug. In fact, if you were to overdose on acetaminophen and were rushed to the emergency room, in an effort to prevent complete liver failure, they would give you N-acetylcysteine (NAC), an amino acid known to immediately boost the production of glutathione.

The study below surmises that the association of serum GGT with type 2 diabetes reflects an exposure to environmental toxins (they postulate persistent organic pollutants as the toxin). Why? Because it is a well-known fact that persistent organic pollutants, which reside in fat tissue, behave as endocrine disruptors as seen in diabetes and inflammation. It is also a well-known statistic that most diabetics are overweight (especially type 2 diabetics).

> The results of several epidemiological studies of serum gamma-glutamyltransferase (an enzyme that catalyzes the reaction between a peptide and an amino acid) (GGT) led us to hypothesize that associations of GGT within its normal range with type 2 diabetes may reflect detrimental effects of **xenobiotics** found in the environment, such as **persistent organic pollutants** (POPs). [Lee DH et al Can persistent organic pollutants explain the association between serum gamma-glutamyltransferase and type 2 diabetes? *Diabetologia* 2008 Mar;51(3):402-7.]

Are You Confused?

Nearly every day you will hear some news release about how certain supplements are detrimental or don't work. In May, 2008, the news was how taking antioxidants can cause death if taken during cancer treatment. Are you confused? I've been hearing both sides of every health, medical and nutrition story for over 40 years. I've learned to always look at it from God's point of view.

What is God's point of view with regard to antioxidants. Are antioxidants detrimental? Absolutely not, and quite the contrary. Without them we would *die* a quick and painful death from the attack of oxygen free radicals and other toxins upon our cells. They are so important in fact, that God in His wisdom saw fit to make nearly every vitamin, mineral, amino acid and food compound participate in some way in antioxidant activity! In fact, scientists are still counting the various antioxidants found in foods – at last count there are over 6,000 antioxidant compounds within the phytochemical category of "phenols" alone!

While you cannot see those antioxidants busily standing guard at your cells, protecting you from grave harm, they *are* there. I had one experience with anitoxidants that forever changed me. I went to the dentist for the major dentistry which I describe in Chapter 6 *Dental Work*. I had been told to consume nothing from midnight on as I'd be given conscious sedation. I did as I was told, was given the sedation, was asleep within minutes and the extractions proceeded. I awoke hours later. I went home and recuperated and about three weeks later returned for some more work that I was told would only require local anesthesia. That morning I didn't eat, but I took my usual supplements, which were a handful of antioxidants, including 500 mg. of Vitamin C. It turned out I needed the sedation after all to prepare another tooth for a crown. I was given the same medication I'd taken the first time which had knocked me out in minutes. This time, over an hour later I was still wide awake.

It was the vitamin C! This was a major lightbulb moment, because there had been many times I'd gone to the dentist and the anesthesia didn't work well and I was given multiple injections and suffered much pain until they could finally anesthetize me. On more than one occasion the injections exceeded a dozen shots and reached the limit of what the doctor deemed safe. I recall praying more than once for God to not let me die of so much medication as I began to feel "odd", lightheaded, heart palpitating. I would go home and tell my husband that it was another bad experience where I'd been injected over a dozen times, and that I'd lost count. Now I know to *not* take Vitamin C or other antioxidants *before* going to the dentist, but being prepared to take them all immediately after the appointment. In fact, I'd take it with me, and immediately in the car, I'd take the antioxidant. Vitamin C is a powerful neutralizer of toxins – and anesthesia is definitely a toxin to the body. Smokers and big city dwellers should take 500 mg several times throughout each day!

Antioxidants work, and they work powerfully. So what's this about them causing death if taken during cancer therapies? Consider the toxic nature of the drugs given for cancer therapy. I often wonder if a person merely tolerates those therapies in those times the drugs seem to work, while their own body heals them? I say this because many people who get cancer don't live very long after undergoing extensive cancer therapies. On the other hand, I've known people who drink organic green and carrot juices with or without the toxic drug therapies given for cancer, and have often beat the cancer! So saying that antioxidants cause "death" I believe is highly irresponsible, and any deaths doctors have observed would have occurred anyway from the cancer – not from the antioxidants. However, to explain that antioxidants can neutralize some of the toxic effects of the therapies would be far more truthful.

So *don't* be confused. Look at everything from Nature and God's viewpoint and not man's. There's a reason for the saying, "the wisdom of man is foolishness". Man slants things in his favor with regard to his bank account, his reputation, his "status", and his ego...neither God nor Nature will lie to you for their own gain.

Avoiding All Pollutants In General

Anything cleaved from its natural place in Nature (such as when we isolate, hydrolyze, ferment or texturize proteins) or concentrated (such as when we extract sugar from fruits to make that concentrated deadly white powder) or otherwise denatured and then added to our foods, is nearly always, in some way, to some degree, dangerous. If you are seeking health, or trying to keep the health you have, you must stick to pure, whole foods. When you choose your diet it is by far easier and wiser to simply choose whole foods to which nothing has been added than to read lengthy "ingredients". If there are 20+ ingredients in a food, and if you can't pronounce or define even just *one* of those ingredients, don't choose that "food".

Choose what you *can* have, rather than focus on what you cannot. The list of foods with additives that are contradictory to good health is enormous. But if you find for some reason you must consume a food with a "list of ingredients", by all means read each and every one, and make sure, above all, there are no glutamate sources (go to www.truthinlabeling.org or email questions to adandjack@aol.com or call (858) 481-9333). Again, if a food has an extensive list of ingredients, the chances are quite high that many of those ingredients are not conducive to good health or healing.

For example, I wrote to "Jack" at truthinlabeling with a question I've had for years. "Why is 'citric acid' on the glutamate list, isn't it 'vitamin C'?" He answered:

"Vitamin C is ascorbic acid, not citric acid. In past years citric acid came from citrus fruits, such as the lemons. However, currently most of the citric acid on the market is made from corn. When producing the citric acid from corn, producers do not take the time nor expend the money to remove all protein. The remaining protein is broken down, at least in part, resulting in some processed free glutamic acid (MSG). There still is some pure citric acid on the market, but it is rarely found." [Jack Samuels truthinlabeling.org adandjack@aol.com]

Jump ahead a few months. I was at Marie Callender's for dinner with a large group of family before going to see one of our talented kids in a musical performance. It was also just a day after my husband's birthday. I had the usual salad bar, and only used plain oil and vinegar on the salad. But I decided I'd have the raspberry ice tea – to *celebrate the birthday*. I'd had raspberry ice tea a couple of times elsewhere without any problem. Mind you, I'm now at the point on this health journey, where I don't take chances at all – but this time I goofed. Within hours I felt as if I was under water, my eardrums felt pressurized, there was a swooshing in my ears, and my hearing was less than half normal. But worse, it felt as if I had a brain aneurysm that could burst at any moment. I felt awful, and it was frightening.

Had this happened years ago I would have been clueless. But this time, I *immediately* thought: *the raspberry tea!* I relate this so you might understand sooner rather than later, that you must never assume — for example, that raspberry tea that is just herbal tea, perhaps with a bit of sugar added at one restaurant, is the same at another. I spent the entire night feeling like I was once again, "done with life". The misery was just too much. I came home from the show and took eight activated charcoal tablets with a glass of water. I took extra CaAEP by the method explained in section 15 "When You Can't Take A Supplement Orally", Chapter 11. Then I lay awake, miserable until I fell asleep, exhausted at 3:00 a.m.

The next day my ears were still pressurized and the hearing still about half of normal. I drove over to Marie Callender's and told them I needed to see the ingredients on the raspberry ice tea to check if I could have it (told them I had "allergies"). They kindly dug the label out of the trash and brought it to me. *There were two sources of free glutamates in it.* Now here's where we *really* need to know even the so-called "potential" sources. The truth is, if there are ingredients in anything that *may* have free glutamates, its about 99.9% assured that it *does* have free glutamates. There's just no need to be so mysterious like saying "natural flavorings" or "seasonings", etc. The main source of free glutamates in that tea was "citric acid". (See text box above.) Even without the citric acid and "natural flavorings", the tea was basically sugar water (high fructose corn syrup, a highly refined sugar, not compatible with health) and chemicals. A label that should have read water, herb tea and sugar actually had about 20 ingredients, mostly chemicals.

Avoiding Glutamates

Keep in mind that the three pollutants you need to focus upon avoiding are: mercury, glutamates and pesticides, and when you strictly avoid *them* you will often automatically be avoiding many other chemicals as well.

Let's consider just glutamates, most often thought of as "MSG" (although it is hidden in over 40 substances). First of all, if there is a *suspicion* of a food containing MSG, then believe it does and *do not* consume it. The tons of glutamates being added to foods is real, and devastating – far more than anyone realizes. Go to www.truthinlabeling.org and avoid all the names that are absolutely MSG as well as all those that "may contain" glutamates. It's my experience that if they "may" contain – they *do.* Early on in my glutamate education I wanted a "treat", so I put a little parmesan cheese on my vegetables. I got a whopping migraine. I looked at the label, it said "enzymes". Turns out the enzymes break down the protein in the cheese and generate free glutamates. I don't eat anything with enzymes anymore because it *may* (and likely *does*) have free glutamates.

"In hundreds of studies around the world, scientists were creating **obese** mice and rats to use in diet or diabetes test studies. No strain of rat or mice is naturally obese, so the scientists have to create them. They make these morbidly obese creatures by injecting them with MSG when they are first born. The **MSG triples the amount of insulin the pancreas creates**; causing rats (and humans?) to become obese. They even have a title for the fat rodents they create: "MSG-Treated Rats". I was shocked too. I went to my kitchen, checking the cupboards and the fridge. MSG was in everything: The Campbell's soups, the Hostess Doritos [sic], the Lays flavored potato chips, Top Ramen, Betty Crocker Hamburger Helper, Heinz canned gravy, Swanson frozen prepared meals, Kraft salad dressings, especially the 'healthy low fat' ones. The items that didn't have MSG marked on the product label had something called "Hydrolyzed Vegetable Protein", which is just another name for Monosodium Glutamate." [Robban Sica, MD Center for the Healing Arts in Orange, Connecticut]

Glutamates Are Deadly, And Added To Most Processed Foods

Glutamates are far more involved in disease than you realize, *especially* after mercury has damaged your glutamatergic system (in essence, the system using glutamates that "fires" your neurons allowing them to synapse and do their job).

"This MSG story, which I have known about for years, is FAR WORSE than (just causing obesity). The truth is MSG directly increases glutamate levels and directly in the presence of calcium leads to CELL DEATH. (This affects) Memory, Alzheimer's, ADHD and all of Neurobiology." [Garry F. Gordon MD,DO,MD(H) President, Gordon Research Institute]

You may find glutamates interchangeably discussed as MSG, excitotoxins, glutamic acid, and monosodium glutamate. You need to also know that free glutamates are a *part* of not just 25, but over 40 other food additives as obscure as "natural flavoring" or "seasonings" (if they don't tell you exactly *what* seasonings, its often because they are hiding MSG). In addition, aspartate is the other common excitotoxin not often mentioned, but also needs to be avoided. Consumed on a daily basis, glutamates will eventually cause continuing damage because they cause neurons to fire out of control, and die. Glutamates powerfully affect the course of a disease and promote rapid worsening. Again, there are so many "things going on" in all diseases that people can easily be confused. Remember that mercury damages the glutamatergic system first, which then cannot handle the copious amount of free glutamate consumed daily.

The Far-Reaching Damage Done By Glutamates

1. In the quest to understand the mechanisms of diabetes because of its unprecedented rise in children, it was learned that roughly 85% of those studied with **Type 1 diabetes** had antibodies against **glutamic acid.** In addition, MSG causes a very large insulin response after it is ingested since there are glutamate receptors in the pancreas. [M Solimena et al. *NEJM* Vol 322:1555-1560 May 31, 1990 No. 22.]

2. **Glutamate** uses the same transport system as cysteine, taurine's metabolic precursor, hence glutamate competes for

uptake with the amino acid the body uses to make taurine. This could result in **MSG overload** causing taurine deficiency. Taurine deficiency is involved in **epilepsy, vision problems, atrial fibrillation**, and **blood pressure problems.** [http://www.msgtruth.org/diabetes.htm]

3. Blood vessel vasodilation and inflammation are implicated in **migraines** and one of the actions of glutamate is vasodilation plus factors that lead to inflammation. [It was found that glutamate, a major neurotransmitter, is vasoactive in the cerebral circulation. Glutamate-induced cerebral arteriolar dilation. [Wei Meng, MD et al. Glutamate-Induced Cerebral Vasodilation Is Mediated by Nitric Oxide Through N-Methyl-D-Aspartate Receptors. *Stroke.* 1995;26:857-863.]

4. Decreased Levels of dopamine have been recently linked to **ADHD. Glutamate** in animal studies decreased dopamine. [Glutamate produced a concentration-dependent decrease in extracellular dopamine. Matthew T. Taber et al. **Glutamate receptor agonists decrease extracellular dopamine in the rat nucleus accumbens in vivo.** Correspondence to Hans C. Fibiger, Division of Neurological Sciences, Department of Psychiatry, University of British Columbia, 2255 Wesbrook Mall, Vancouver, B.C. V6T 1ZS, Canada.]

5. There is new research that points specifically to **MSG** as a factor in both **ADHD** and **autism** - both unheard of before 1950. According to new research from Johns Hopkins, the immune system is distressed by nervous system over-stimulation. MSG is a nervous system *excitotoxin,* causing neurons to fire excessively. [Search for: *Food Additive Excitotoxins and Degenerative Brain Disorders* by Russell L. Blaylock, MD or: http://www.jpands.org/hacienda/article27.html]

6. **Glutamate** has been shown to **increase histamine** by 150%. Since glutamate triggers a more severe histamine response than otherwise would be suffered by the people with **allergies** (for example to peanuts) while **MSG** may not kill

the highly allergic directly, it can most definitely act as an accomplice. [Nitric oxide-induced glutamate release seems to exert a subordinate stimulatory effect on histamine release. Helmut Prast et al. *Naunyn-Schmiedeberg's Archives of Pharmacology* Volume 354, Number 6, December, 1996]

7. Abnormally high levels of **glutamate** have been found in the cerebrospinal fluid (the clear watery fluid that surrounds the brain and the spinal cord) of some patients with **ALS** [Lou Gehrig's Disease]. http://www.fda.gov/fdac/features/796_als.html]

Amyotrophic lateral sclerosis (ALS) is a progressive neurological disorder characterised by degeneration of upper and lower motor neurons. Whilst the primary pathogenic trigger is unknown in most cases, evidence is mounting to implicate a role for **glutamate-mediated neurotoxicity** in the disorder. [*J Neurol* 1999 Dec;246(12):1140-4.]

---

8. Laboratory animals fed **MSG** have been found to develop **damage to the retina of the eye**, where there are **glutamate** receptors. [The first published report of human adverse reactions to "processed free glutamic acid" was by Kwok, R.H.M. The Chinese restaurant syndrome. Letter to the editor. *N Engl J Med* 278: 796, 1968. That report had been preceded by published studies demonstrating that processed free glutamic acid caused retinal degeneration. www.truthinlabeling.org]

9. MSG also affects the **cardiovascular** system because glutamate is a calcium channel opener and affects vascular constriction. ["Subsequent studies have shown that glutamate, and other excitatory amino acids, attach to a specialized family of receptors (NMDA, kainate, AMPA and metabotrophic) which in turn, either directly or indirectly, opens the calcium channel on the neuron cell membrane, allowing calcium to flood into the cell." *Food Additive Excitotoxins*

and Degenerative Brain Disorders by Russell L. Blaylock, MD or: http://www.jpands.org/hacienda/article27.html]

10. The results of putting both pets and people on **glutamate/ aspartate restricted diets** have been no less than *astounding*, not only for **epilepsy** but also for **autism, insomnia, pain, ADHD,** and even **MS** and **ALS**. [http://www.dogtorj.com/ or search for: Dogtorj]

11. A recent research press release from Johns Hopkins linked *nervous system stimulation* to the immune response and **asthma** in particular. They don't say that glutamate stimulates the nervous system — *but that's exactly what it does.* [Also see: Monosodium L-glutamate-induced asthma. Allen DH - *J Allergy Clin Immunol* — October 1, 1987; 80(4): 530-7]

12. **According to the following study, beta amyloid protein deposits in the brain seen in Alzheimer's disease actually increase the neurotoxicity of glutamate in the brain.** [http://www.jneurosci.org/cgi/content/abstract/12/2/376. **Neuron (nerve cell) death** is due to the **neurotoxic effects of excess glutamate** in the brain.]

13. It is not surprising that **MSG** also **affects hearing** considering that glutamate is what the hair cell in the ear uses as a neurotransmitter. **Ringing in the ears** is a common complaint of **MSG** sufferers. [Nearly 90 percent of a small group of people with tinnitus reported substantial relief after taking the drug acamprosate. The researchers attributed acamprosate's success to its effect on glutamate, an amino acid that stimulates activity of the nervous system. Their theory is that tinnitus is caused by disruptions in **the same glutamate pathways that are involved in addiction to alcohol.** **Search for: Acamprosate ringing in the ears.**]

14. "Researchers have observed abnormally high levels of **glutamate** in people and animals with **glaucoma**. Glutamate is an amino acid that excites nerve cells. In the eye this occurs during vision. Some experts theorize that in glaucoma, either reduced blood flow or increased pressure on nerve cells

triggers the release of excess glutamate. In large amounts, glutamate causes the nerve cells to fire intensively, which eventually destroys them." [University of Maryland Medical Center. Http://www.umm.edu/patiented/articles/what_causes_glaucoma_optic_nerve_damage_000025_2.htm]

The list goes on and on. MSG, glutamate, aspartate, excitotoxins, monosodium glutamate as well as 40 other chemical compounds that *contain* free glutamates are routinely added to foods and are highly *deleterious*. For people who get migraines from ingesting any amount of MSG, the excrutiating pain is their motivation to know where free glutamates exist so they can be completely avoided. But the danger is just as real to everyone else wanting to preserve their eyesight, their hearing, their brain. It's almost too bad that everyone doesn't get migraines so they'll be motivated to completely eliminate glutamates before its too late.

Brain Lesions Caused By Glutamates

The Journal of Neural Transmission, January, 2006 (p. 102-110) reports on how "excitotoxic over-stimulation" (although they blame it on "excess release of excitatory neurotransmitter glutamate" while completely ignoring the tons of free glutamates people consume daily) leads to "**glutamate lesions**". While there is no question that glutamates damage white matter, it is *mercury* that damages the glutamatergic system, leading to glutamate's excess and ability to damage white matter.

I personally have done a Tesla MRI (2006) and found "white matter lesions" on my brain in the exact spot from which my migraines have always eminated. What the above-referenced study is saying, is that an excess over-stimulation of glutamate release leads to increases in intracellular calcium levels (not good), over-activation of different protein kinases and triggering enzyme reactions which finally result in excessive production of oxygen free radicals (like nitric oxide) all of which does *damage to cell membranes and ultimately causes neuronal death*. And this neuronal death, depending upon where and how bad, is what leads to the various neurological diseases like migraines, but also Alzheimer's, Parkinson's, multiple sclerosis, autism and more.

In 2008 the *Journal of Autoimmunity* reported on studies done on MSG. Researchers from the Department of Diagnostic Pathology, Graduate School of Medicine and Pharmaceutical Sciences, University of Toyama, Japan discovered that glutamate (MSG) causes chronic inflammation leading to autoimmune diseases, liver cancer, obesity and type 2 diabetes. With grave concern, and in light of the fact that metric tons of free glutamates are added to food supplies worldwide, they recommended that MSG should have its safety profile quickly re-examined, and likely withdrawn, as they said, "from the food chain." What a dream come true that would be for me! (And for you, even if you don't realize it.) If I could focus on only two or three things the rest of my life, one would be to create a world without the use of free glutamates. I guarantee that it would rid the world of untold pain and neurological destruction free glutamates cause.

People can go most of their life consuming high levels of free glutamates and not know the damage that is brewing internally. By the time the hearing is gone, the eyesight is dimmed or the brain has white matter lesions, the suffering has been enormous, and turning around the disease process would be insurmountable for most people. Of course its never *too* late, and once you know the truth you *must* try to turn things around. So true is the saying, "where there's breath, there's life" (and thus hope). But first, of course, we must each stop being poisoned by mercury in every way we can.

Mercury Caused The Initial Damage

When cells are injured they release **substance P** [a protein substance that stimulates nerve endings increasing <u>pain</u> messages]; *and* **CGRP** [Calcitonin-gene-related peptide – a neuropeptide with strong <u>vasodilating</u> action as seen in migraines and other pain]. But when cells are injured, they also release **glutamate** [a neurotransmitter protein whose main job it is to "<u>excite</u>" neurons into synapsing (synapse - the junction between two nerve cells across which a nerve impulse is transmitted)].

When injury is severe (as when there is mercury damage) and/ or ongoing (as in consuming copious quantities of free glutamates like we do daily in the typical American diet) the repeated release of substance P, CGRP and glutamate causes changes in the **nociceptive neurons** ("pain perceiving" neurons) which become chronically **hyperexcitable**. Now, even the smallest provocations can spark this vicious cycle of releasing substance P, CGRP and glutamate. For those whose bodies and brains have been damaged by mercury, this means chronic neurological injury and pain caused and worsened by glutamate consumption, alcohol, estrogen fluctuations, insulin (sugar consumption) and more.

Recent studies have indicated that **insulin activates endothelial nitric-oxide synthase** (eNOS) by protein kinase B (PKB)-mediated phosphorylation at Ser^{1177} in endothelial cells. [Note: Nitric oxide is made from endothelial nitric-oxide synthase] [J. Biol. Chem., Vol. 278, Issue 21, 18791-18797, May 23, 2003]

When there is repeated release of glutamate, this results in the prolonged opening of **post-synaptic ion channels** [post-synaptic just means where two nerves are sending messages from one to the other, and where they connect (the synapse), the "post" is the "other side". Think of it as neuron "a" and neuron "b", "post" is on the "b" side.] Prolonged opening of the ion channels causes an influx of calcium and sodium into the cells and thus an outpouring of inflammatory **arachidonic acid** (inflammatory fatty acid). An ion channel is a protein that acts as a hole or opening in a cell membrane and permits the selective entrance or exit of ions (like potassium, sodium, and calcium). These ions act as electrical currents passing in and out of the cell. Ion channels are critical in the healthy functioning of cells in many ways, not the least of which is the regulation of everything within the cell that is supposed to stay within, and keeping out of the cell everything that is supposed to stay out – or at least a balancing of each at any given time.

When there is an assault on your cells there is a resultant **vasoconstriction** (your blood vessels constrict or shrink down as if to stop the flow of toxic blood – well known in cardiovascular (e.g., angina) and other diseases). Think of it this way, if someone attacks you, you "shrink back" from the attack. Your cells and blood vessels do similarly. This vasoconstriction likely accounts for the "aura" some migraineurs get, or the fatigue in MS among other symptoms that would follow a lack of blood flow throughout the body.

Along comes **nitric oxide** to "mediate" the assault. Nitric oxide is a well-known **vasodilator.** But excessive assault and vasoconstriction can and does lead to excessive nitric oxide production, especially in people whose glutamatergic system is damaged by mercury.

Researchers believe that **nitric oxide** (NO) forms in neurons following a series of molecular reactions that occur in a matter of milliseconds. Many of the specifics of NO production are still unclear. For example, it's not known how often NO is produced or how involved different participants need to be in order to carry out the production. It's thought that the molecule **glutamate** can start the process by leaving a neuron and attaching to a molecule lining an adjacent neuron, known as the NMDA receptor (a type of glutamate receptor). Their union causes calcium molecules to enter the receiving cell. This can trigger the activation of the enzyme NOS, which synthesizes nitric oxide. Some researchers believe that nitric oxide production normally aids brain function, but **overproduction of the gas can kill neurons.** [Journal of Neuroscience, Vol 13, 2651-2661, 1993.]

The truth is, we will find nitric oxide being implicated in many inflammatory, neurological and chronic pain diseases because the body produces it in response to injury! When the glutamatergic system has been damaged, this has been shown to eventually lead to the production of excitotoxic glutamate at the slightest provocation which will then be accompanied by a similar toxic level of nitric oxide.

Nitric oxide (NO) mediates several biological actions, including relaxation of blood vessels. **NO mediates the neurotoxicity of glutamate.** [*Proc. Natl. Acad. Sci. USA* Vol. 88, pp. 6368-6371, July 1991 Neurobiology.]

Researchers and writers will point to the presence of nitric oxide in migraines, multiple sclerosis, Parkinson's, Alzheimer's, ALS, and more wondering if it *causes* the disease. The answer is no. Once again, *mercury* caused the initial injury that led to a long series of events that involve excess glutamate release which causes excess nitric oxide release in response to the cellular assault and injury. No mercury = None of these diseases.

> Evidence that **nitric oxide** plays an important role in **multiple sclerosis** is accumulating rapidly. Certainly nitric oxide is produced within the inflammatory lesions, in MS, seemingly in relatively high concentrations, and it has potent effects on immune and excitable cells. [Multiple Sclerosis as a Neuronal Disease by Stephen G. Waxman. Published by Academic Press, 2005 ISBN 0127387617 496 pages]

In Stephen Waxman's book, he rightfully points out that we now know that MS is more than just a demylenating disorder, and that MS affects more than just the white matter. He says, and rightfully so: *neurons are injured in MS*. The truth is, *mercury* injured those neurons and we have the film produced by some brilliant researchers in Canada to prove it.

You Can Stop Being Poisoned By Mercury

The three steps you can take immediately to stop ingesting mercury is:

1. **No amalgam fillings** ever again. As your fillings need replacing, replace with white fillings. If you can afford to take amalgams out, you can do so, but find a dentist who uses all the proper precautions when doing so.
2. **Don't eat fish.** Our waters are toxic, fish are full of mercury. The exceptions are so rare, that it's safest just to not eat fish at all.
3. **No immunizations.** You don't really need them anyway. What you *need* is a strong immune system. Work instead on that. If you feel the need for immunizations, make the doctor prove

to you that the injection does not contain mercury or any other toxic ingredient, like aluminum (common) or formaldehyde. These might be hidden by manufacturer's names (for example, the mercury is called thimerosal).

Please don't do as many people do when you hear another news report that tells you about yet another toxin. Don't exclaim "everything" is toxic, as an excuse to not even try. When you hear, for example, that there are toxic phthalates in plastic, and the recommendation is to not drink water out of plastic bottles or cook in the microwave with plastic, simply stop using plastic in those ways. You will be rewarded for your efforts! Buy organic! Avoid anything and everything that is a man-made chemical and therefore likely toxic. Use natural products. It's actually a fun challenge to do as much as you can. Tell yourself, "The number of toxins are many and complicated, but the answer, to stick to God-made foods and products, is simple." You'll be doing your body, your children's body, and the entire world a favor.

Focus On The Prevalent Three: Mercury, Glutamates And Pesticides

If you're feeling helpless or hopeless, don't. You can take powerful and effective steps in eliminating the three most prevalent pollutants from your body and environment. Concern yourself with mercury (no more immunizations, amalgams or seafood), pesticides (buy organic foods) and glutamates (consume nothing seasoned by others, and/or get the list of possible glutamate sources and read labels carefully). These are given the emphasis because they are the *most* prevalent, affect *everyone* on a daily basis, and are the main culprits in neurological diseases. Of course you want to eliminate *all* toxic metals, and as you continue on your journey, you will naturally become aware of them, and where they exist so you can make sure you have no contact with them.

Of course there are other toxic food additives, but again, glutamates are the worst and most prevalent on the list. Glutamates are found in altered, fermented, hydrolyzed and isolated protein products. You will find that as you eliminate glutamates, you will naturally eliminate other toxic amines. This is because the same foods that have been fermented or processed to generate the free glutamates (like all fermented soy and wheat products — miso, soy sauce, tamari, etc.) will logically have other altered proteins making them unhealthful to the human body.

Mercury has been documented to cause **autoimmune disease** and many researchers have concluded that autoimmunity is a factor in the major chronic neurological diseases such as **multiple sclerosis, Lou Gehrig's disease, Parkinson's disease, systemic lupus erythematosus, rheumatoid arthritis,** etc. Mercury and other toxic metals also form inorganic compounds with OH, NH2, CL, in addition to the SH radical and thus inhibits many cellular enzyme processes, coenzymes, hormones, and blood cells. Mercury has been found to impair conversion of thyroid T4 hormone to the active T3 form as well as causing autoimmune thyroiditis common to such patients. In general, immune activation from toxic metals such as mercury resulting in cytokine release and abnormalities of the hypothalamus-pituitary-adrenal (HPA) axis can cause changes in the brain, fatigue, and severe psychological symptoms such as profound fatigue, musculoskeletal pain, sleep disturbances, gastrointestinal and neurological problems as are seen in CFS, fibromyalgia, and autoimmune thyroiditis. [Bernard Windham(Ed.)

In the chapters on psoriasis, migraines and multiple sclerosis, as well as the chapter on Nature's medicines, you will find personal experience along with the science relating how I acquired all the diseases from which I now suffer *and* how there are many nutritional, herbal, and natural therapies, that can keep you "humming along" to where life can be rich and full. My hope is that you will extract the truths that can help you prevent suffering as well as understand your own suffering. In writing this, instead of getting bogged down in thinking I have to list copious references (as if to impress), possibly resulting in never getting this information to you (or worse, boring you to death),

I endeavored to keep it simple, and leave it to *you* to continue in your journey of seeking the truth – by going to various informational websites (those seeking only the truth) such as www.pubmed.gov or www.mercola.com or www.lef.org or www.truthinlabeling.org.

I'm clearly not doing my job if I can't help you realize that your own country, your own doctor or dentist may very well be causing your (or a family member's) suffering, pain, devastation, loss of income, loss of security, loss of hope for a future and joy. Unfortunately most people still believe that they were walking along, minding their own business, and a disease bug came out of nowhere and "bit" them. I also think that most people still believe that you can go to a doctor or dentist and they'll know exactly what you have and how to fix you. Of course *neither of these is true* according to my experience of over 30 years in the medical and alternative medical field, observing thousands of people, their illnesses, and outcomes, as well as with my own health issues.

Today, one in every two people are coming down with a devastating disease. The type of disease a person gets, and the severity, depends upon the level and duration of toxic exposure. A simple concept, really – but one that seems to go right over the heads of most people. The worst of the toxins by both quantity and level of toxicity are **mercury, glutamates and pesticides.** Emerging rapidly as the fourth pollutant by virtue of prevalence now is **radiation** from cell phones, computers, "wi-fi" etc. That would be the subject of an entire book of its own. Suffice it to say here that both lessening their use and *distance* from your cell phone, cathode ray TV or computer screen, and of course x-rays, is your best prevention.

God gave humans and animals the intelligence and ability to eat right, get sunshine, exercise, drink pure water, rest and *get well.* Doctors, often take *away* that ability to get well by applying one toxic measure after another.

Chapter 4
PARASITES TAKE OVER

Chronic disease occurs at that point when pollutants have damaged cells of the gut, internal organs, metabolic and immune systems all to the point where the process of inflammation is chronic, and parasites can now invade these damaged and weak cells, tissues and organs, and *feast* upon them largely unopposed.

Opportunistic Parasites

Parasites that normally exist in your body and environment are mostly merely opportunistic, entering and damaging your cells, tissues and organs only when your defenses are down. Parasites are organisms that live in or on and take nourishment from another organism. This includes viruses, fungi, bacteria and worms. Yes, humans get worms! And yes, a virus is a parasite. Normally, your body is designed to fight parasites. But when your defenses are damaged irreparably by pollutants, the parasites can invade unopposed. God didn't create you, born with all you need to breathe, eat, eliminate, attack foreign invaders, smile, laugh, love and live, to get Parkinson's, multiple sclerosis, asthma, psoriasis, cancer, or Lou Gehrig's disease – yet *more than half* of us are getting diseases like these. So how is this happening, and in such epidemic proportions? The answer is simple but true, and worth repeating until we all fully understand: **Pollutants** damage your cells; **Parasites** opportunistically invade your cells, take up residence, do great damage; and **Nutritional Deficiencies** make healing even more difficult if not impossible.

What Are Parasites?

A parasite, as we said above, by definition feeds off of a host. You are the host. Actually, more accurately, any of your 10-100 trillion cells are the host. Parasites do not feed off healthy tissue, they seek out damaged, diseased and dying tissue, such as that which has been damaged by pollutants and unprotected by antioxidants and other nutrients.

Bacteria

Everyone knows about bacteria because every time you go to the doctor and you're not feeling well he/she will prescribe an antibiotic. What most people don't know even today, is that *most* bacteria are actually "good", meaning they do a lot of good things in the world and your body, like consuming bad bacteria, or breaking down foods for digestion. What most people also still don't know even today, is that giving antibiotics for every infection is a common contributing factor to death by doctor/hospital.

This is from a "Yahoo" question/answer online:

Antibiotics do compromise the immune system and that leaves you open to many other infectious diseases. After 5 months of taking antibiotics, your immune system must be completely trashed. There are over 400 species of bacteria and yeast which inhabit the intestinal tract. These "Good Bacteria" help keep potentially harmful bacteria and yeast in check. Probiotics should be used while taking antibiotics (my note: don't take at same time). [http://answers.yahoo.com/question/index?qid=20080711135759AATIERT]

So true, and if you hear or read anyone saying that antibiotics don't harm your immune system (even your doctor) *they are blatantly wrong.* Here's what science says:

Although there are several lines of evidence for a prompt use of antibiotics in life-threatening infections, restricting the use of antibiotics should remain the common rule. Good evidence suggests that a strategy aiming at reducing the prolonged use of broad-spectrum antibiotics is the only means to reduce the emergence of multiresistant bacteria. [*Curr Opin Crit Care* 2008 Oct;14(5):587-92.]

The problem will be greatly magnified if you use antibiotics in a body already damaged by mercury as well. You will find that the presence of an overgrowth of both fungus and viruses will be exacerbated to a painful or even deadly degree. Bacteria, viruses and fungus in a healthy body, not damaged by mercury, don't really have much hope of replicating (which as you will see below, is a virus' only "purpose" in life).

Abigail Salyers is a microbiologist researching good bacteria and how they go bad. She says they do this by exchanging a little DNA and then moving on to their next encounter. One alarming thing she has found in her many years of study is that the bacterial cells don't even need to touch to exchange the DNA. One way they can do it is by bursting, and their contents are released into the surrounding area and taken up by other bacteria. Why do they do this? One reason is to survive.

This is where antibiotics come in. When antibiotics are given for every little sniffle and sneeze, bacteria "modify" themselves to survive against antibiotics. Ms. Salyers is part of a team of researchers and healthcare professionals who fear that these antibiotic-resistent strains of bacteria are quickly becoming a world-wide threat. If the bacteria win we will see people dying from routine medical procedures, as well as from aggressive skin infections. We will see a rise in fatalities from what used to be "routine" infections, easily handled by antibiotics, like urinary tract or heart infections. Salyers warns that the flagrant use of antibiotics must stop.

In addition, the U.S. Food and Drug Administration says that 70% of bacteria that causes infections in hospitals are now resistant to at least one antibiotic routinely used to fight them. They also tell us that 41% of strep infections are now resistant to penicillin. The list goes on. What's the answer? The answer is a super healthy immune system, and reserving your use of antibiotics for that one infection in your life when it is life-threatening. Honestly, most people could go their entire life never needing antibiotics. There are so many powerful dietary and supplemental things that can be done to boost the immune system and even directly destroy bacterial infections. See Chapter 11 *Nature's Medicines.*

Viruses

Viruses can only survive by getting either themselves, or their genetic material inside of your cells so they can replicate. Antibiotics do nothing to destroy viruses, mostly because the virus hides within your cells. A virus has genes made of DNA or RNA which is what it uses to make copies of itself. But again, it must do so inside of your cells. When a virus enters your cells, this is the point at which you are said to be "infected". The sole purpose of most viruses are to make copies of themselves. When they do so, they take over the cell they inhabit and their replication leads to the death of that cell.

Every species of man, animal and plant may have 100 or more different viruses which can infect that species. Plant viruses will only infect plants. Animal viruses will only infect animals and human viruses will only infect humans.

Humans are protected from viruses by a couple of different means. First a viral infection can lead to the synthesis and secretion of substances called *interferons*. These proteins interact with adjacent cells which help adjacent cells become more resistant to infection by the virus. Sometimes, this resistance isn't quite good enough to prevent the spread of the virus to more and more cells, and we begin to feel sick. It is at that point you will know you have "an infection". *If your body's immune system is intact*, it will take over and start to fight the infection by killing the virus on the outside of the cells but will also kill infected cells in an attempt to protect you. Of course, the killing of the infected cells prevents the spread of the virus, since a virus requires a living cell in order for the virus to be able to replicate. Eventually, the viruses can be greatly lessened in numbers, and you can get over the symptoms they are causing. So far as we know, once you have a virus living within you, you will have it the rest of your life. If your immune system and other cells have been damaged by pollutants, viruses can have easier and continuous access to your cells, causing frequent infections and widespread damage to your body, such as that seen with herpes involvement in various diseases like multiple sclerosis and cancer.

HIV is an exception to this situation because HIV infects cells of the immune system which are necessary to kill the infected cells. HIV itself does not directly cause "AIDS", but the eventual death of immune cells due to infection with the human immunodeficiency virus (HIV) allows other infections to ultimately harm and even cause the death of the host.

Fungus

It is actually quite common to have a fungal infection. Fungal infections are so common, in fact, that most doctors don't even bother to test for them unless there are massive outward signs (like thrush in the mouth). This is too bad, because like so many other things we consider "normal", having an overgrowth of fungus is *not* normal, and contributes greatly to disease and suffering. I asked to be tested once, and the doctor flat out refused, saying: "I'd put a swabbing of your saliva, for example, on a petri dish and culture it, and I'd find fungus. I'd find that in everyone."

He said this, as if his findings wouldn't mean anything. But in the doctor's defense, your *symptoms* are a better indication of a problematic level of fungus. However, symptoms of candida (fungus) overgrowth can be the symptoms of other parasitic overgrowths as well. The way to deal with a fungal overgrowth is first by not using antibiotics unless a matter of life or death; by not consuming alcohol or "fiberless sugars" which feed fungus; by eating fresh, raw garlic daily until parasitic symptoms go away; and by consuming a pure, whole, fresh, (preferably organic) mostly plant-based diet.

> Garlic has been shown to inhibit the growth of a variety of microorganisms, not only bacteria but also fungi and viruses. The antimicrobial activity of garlic is believed to be due to the effect of allicin, the main ingredient in garlic, generated by the phosphopyridoxal enzyme allinase. [*Applied And Environmental Microbiology*, Mar. 1987, p. 615-617]

Most "yeast infections" are caused by fungi of the genus *Candida*. Although members of the genus *Candida* continue to be the most common agents of yeast infections, mostly because of the ways in which fungus has been fought medically over the years, yeasts have mutated to where scientists have now described over 200 species of yeasts, in 25 different genre of human infections.

Go to YouTube: http://www.youtube.com/watch?v=ZmHkC2JM53c. "Fungus Eats Man's Face". I watched this years ago, and have been haunted by it ever since, but perhaps for a different reason than you might think. With what I know about God's miraculous gift of our immune system and how people destroy it with mercury, pesticides, smoking, antibiotics, and very poor eating habits, including not getting the nutrients they desperately need for health – what goes through my mind when I think of this man and his wonderful wife is, *it didn't have to happen.*

As an adult human, you have three to four pounds of **beneficial bacteria and yeast** living within your intestines. These microbes compete for nutrients from the food you eat. Usually, the strength in numbers beneficial bacteria enjoy both keeps the ever-present yeasts in check and causes them to produce nutrients such as the B vitamins. However, every time you swallow **antibiotics**, you kill the beneficial bacteria within your intestines. When you do so, you upset the delicate balance of your intestinal terrain. Yeasts grow unchecked into large colonies and take over, in a condition called dysbiosis. [Doug Kaufmann and Dave Holland, MD's "The Fungus Link, Volume 2]

Dysbiosis is a condition wherein the yeast grow into forms that puncture your intestines causing "leaky gut". This in turn sets up a condition wherein macroparticles of food (undigested) can "leak" through the intestinal barrier and into the bloodstream where they are responded to as if they are nasty invaders, or foreigners. The reaction of your body to these invaders involves your immune system responding by launching a cascade of events that can result in any of a number of symptoms that we give names like eczema, psoriasis, allergies, ADHD, hives, headaches and more.

The truth is, when you get a bacterial infection and run for antibiotics, you kill off the beneficial bacteria, and yes, beneficial yeasts that God designed to be your army of fighters against *bad* bacteria and yeasts. These beneficial bacteria help digest food, create nutrients and, again, help protect you from fungus, viruses and bad bacteria. When you're sick, you're supposed to boost your immune system, not destroy it. You boost your immune system with various herbs like echinacea, goldenseal, and grapefruit seed extract; and with vitamins and minerals like vitamin C, bioflavonoids, zinc, selenium; and with various sulfur-rich and polyphenol rich foods like the aforementioned garlic and all fresh (preferably organic) fruits and vegetables. You also boost your immune system by simply going to bed, resting, and drinking lots of pure water to flush your system. Getting out in the sun is another way to boost your immune system! People don't do that anymore! They take pain medications, cold and other medications, and antibiotics, so they can keep running in their hectic lives.

I would *bet* my life that the gentleman who had to have his face entirely removed to eradicate that fungus growing in his sinuses had a very damaged immune system either from excessive antibiotic use or damage from mercury or some other toxin. His fungus was "bread mold" fungus they said. Perhaps he had excessive exposure to that particular fungus. But had he been healthy, it would have been eradicated by a healthy immune system.

There are many "signs" and red flags you can watch for to make sure you don't allow your body to become overburdened with fungus. Here are just a few of the more obvious signs you have a fungal overgrowth. If it is not addressed, all it can do is get worse.

1. Use of antibiotics more than once especially without taking copious amounts of probiotics afterwards
2. Chronic sinus "drip"
3. Coated tongue
4. Excessive consumption or desire for sugar
5. Craving for alcohol
6. "Foggy" feeling in your thinking
7. Fingernails or toenails discolored (white or yellow crusting underneath) lifted away from nailbed (fungus)

A Word About Worms

To learn about worms I will refer you to the fabulous works of Dr. Hulda Regehr Clark who wrote a series of books, one of which is "The Cure for All Cancers". She is perhaps the first brave scientist to come forth with the fact that disease is *caused* by pollutants and parasites. She talks extensively of all bacteria, fungi, viruses and worms. Dr. Clark's emphasis is only slightly different from my own. She emphasizes more of an either/or. Either you're damaged by a pollutant or you're damaged by a parasite. I firmly believe that without the pollutant first, parasites rarely if ever get out of control. Of course there are exceptions to this, like perhaps the HIV virus.

Rediscovering Oxygen – Ozone

I've been using hydrogen peroxide for years. Back in the 1980's I undertook the difficult and painful task of doing hydrogen peroxide I.V.s. At the time there was a man (Keller) in Tijuana who was charging something like $300.00 per session to sit in his roach-infested underground clinic with a hydrogen peroxide IV in your arm for 3-4 hours. I did this at least a dozen times. It wasn't available in the U.S., and I was desperately trying to eradicate my diseases (psoriasis and migraines). I'd read and heard how fabulous oxygen types of therapies are. Well, it was painful, and I don't know that it did much. The worse part was the expense, and the drive down to Tijuana - especially sitting at the border for up to three hours trying to get home at the end of the day. My husband and I went up to 3 times per week for quite some time (he attempting to avoid heart bypass surgery). We spent thousands.

I even purchased all the supplies and did it to myself at home with painfully negative consequences. I never got any embolisms, much less any fatal reaction like the naysayers will warn. What did happen was missing my vein and infusing the hydrogen peroxide into my tissues. It was painful, but nothing more. That's not at all to say that hydrogen peroxide isn't a wonderful thing. Hydrogen peroxide is found in Nature. It is simply water with an extra oxygen. It is a natural, God-given anti-infective. I have continued since the 1980's to always have a bottle of hydrogen peroxide on my sink. I use it to gargle with, put it in the ear for earaches, use to whiten my teeth and more.

In 2007, once again knowing that oxygen is the answer to keep vi-ruses under control – and after suffering since 2004 (after a mercury-riddled hepatitis B shot) with one viral outbreak and symptom after another – I began praying, "*Somewhere* on this planet is *someone* "doing" oxygen to eradicate viruses". I remembered Ed McCabe's book about flooding your body with oxygen, and I ordered it online. When I got the book it was huge and seemed "disjointed" in its writing style. I flipped through it and in an instant decided it was about equipment and clinics and such that I couldn't do. I put it on the shelf for "future reference". At one point months after getting the book I even contem-plated giving it away. But I didn't.

In April of 2008 I went to visit my daughter in Maryland. What a beautiful home she and her husband were able to buy there while he is stationed at a local Naval base. Their backyard is lush and green with many trees and a thick carpet of grass. They have a beautiful deck. I spent a good part of my day sitting in the back yard watching my granddaughter play. The birds sing constantly. Out the front win-dows of their home stretches their lush front lawn, down to a winding cul-de-sac lined with trees. It's this way everywhere in their county. I'd get up in the morning and the sun would be shining, so I'd put on my bathing suit to soak up the sun. Then as the day went on, the sky would cloud over and lightening and rain would come up and we'd rush inside, or home if we were out running errands. Wow! It seemed this happened about every other day!

I was there for almost a week in April, and then returned in June with my husband. We stayed for a week as well. My daughter's hus-band had to go on a trip with his unit for three days. We decided we'd surprise him and paint their large 30x14 foot three level deck. It was badly in need of attention. We went to a local Lowe's, bought the cleaning fluid, the tools, the paint, etc. It was a three day job. All I can tell you is that I looked forward each day to getting up and scrubbing and then painting. I was bending and stretching and kneel-ing and suddenly it hit me! I'd been there about 5 days now and not once did I hurt anywhere, not once did I feel my usual aches and pains in shoulders, back, hips, and head. Although, as I relay in Chapter 8 *Migraines*, after having my root canals out (eliminating a chronic source of infection) I no longer had horrific migraines. But with so much mercury damage, I was still having some aches and pains for which I took Excedrin. But while at my daughter's home, not once did I take an Excedrin.

Now there I was, feeling no need for Excedrin. In fact, I felt 100% wonderful. I was thanking God for how much fun I was having doing that big job. I vowed to continue doing "big jobs" when I got home to California for the accomplishment while benefitting from the exercise and sweating. The first job I could think of was that my own home needed painting.

Then, the day before we were to leave Maryland, that sunny morning we were out running errands, and once again the storm clouds rolled in suddenly. There were distant strikes of lightening, and the wind was coming up. We decided we needed to go home. It was then that I realized what was making me feel so great! Thunderstorms – *ozone.*

I went home and got onto the internet and started doing research. Up came a wonderful video with Ed McCabe – talking about ozone. Go to www.youtube.com and search for "Ed McCabe" or "Mr. Oxygen". Then I remembered that this is what his book was all about. I was anxious to go home and make sure I still had it.

When I got home I researched where the most thunderstorms are, and they're in Florida and up into Maryland...and also in Texas and surrounding areas. They are virtually non-existent in California.

Now I'm thinking...no wonder I can't get control of all my viruses and fungus....there's no ozone here! God gave us ozone to zap parasites and pollutants to keep them under control! I found my copy of Ed McCabe's book, "Flood Your Body With Oxygen" and began to read it. It was all about Ozone. Very interesting now that I was so motivated.

I researched for a few days and then purchased a room Ozonator [from www.Jenesco.com the PRO-4]:

The PRO-4 ozone generator is designed with the professional in mind. It is for use in commercial applications or wherever high ozone output is needed to neutralize stubborn odors, or fight mold and mildew. It is the pro's choice for use in automobiles, limousines, buses, recreational vehicles, rental cars, vans, and boats. It is also excellent for use in hotel and motel rooms, apartments, and extended-stay facilities.

I can't say whether having an ozonator running in your home will get rid of your parasites, and in fact, would say for almost certain it won't by itself. All I know is that ozonated air is one of Nature's gifts among many gifts. I run the ozonator on low an hour on, and half hour off around the clock. My room smells like after a thunderstorm. Ozone isn't a cure-all, but it is a great addition to the many other things you can do for optimal health and minimal pain.

In the future, my hope and prayer for my children and grandchildren is that man wises up and learns to make thorough use of oxygen's powerful healing therapy. It will likely prove to be the only way we can truly rid a body of viruses when no other therapy has ever been found to do so safely.

Endotoxemia

Dr. Henry G. Bieler wrote the book, "Food Is Your Best Medicine". When I was in my 20s I spoke to him on the phone – he was adamant that if "Nature didn't make it, it doesn't belong in the human body". One thing he talked about in his book is how your own gut can manufacture alcohol more "proof" than the strongest alcohol you can buy in a bottle. How? From fermentation in the gut. I personally experienced the truth of what he said so many years ago nearly every time I would eat a dessert on top of a meat meal. That dessert would sit there and ferment horribly and I'd wake up the next day with a "hangover" migraine as if I'd been binge drinking the night before.

When you consume cooked and processed foods, especially grains, sugars and dairy, they will ferment as they slowly pass through the entire length of the digestive tract. In fact, the longer these foods sit in the digestive tract, the more fermentation that can occur. If your digestive system is already damaged by heavy metals, pesticides, antibiotics and other toxins, it is assured you will have a candida (fungal) overgrowth. Because of this, fermentation is simply all the more likely.

The importance of this for people damaged by mercury, migraineurs, people with chronic, painful diseases, and *everybody* is this: Your gut produces alcohol, when you *feed* grains and sugars to the bad bacteria and fungus residing in your gut. The bad bacteria and fungus "ferment" the foods you gave them to "eat" (like using yeast (fungus) to ferment the starch of bread dough. Gas is created and the dough rises). In your gut this fermentation creates alcohol. Alcohol stimulates the production of nitric oxide which leads to migraines, as well as inflammation and disease throughout the body. So whether you drink alcohol, or produce it chronically within your own body (something Dr. Bieler thought most of us do because of our addiction to starches and sugars!) we *end up with nitric oxide.*

Chronic alcohol exposure is reported to increase glutamate-N-methyl-D-aspartate (NMDA) receptors and calcium ion channel activity, resulting in the neurotoxicity and seizure activity associated with alcohol withdrawal in certain persons. Recent information indicates that nitric oxide is responsible for the neurotoxicity associated with excessive glutamate stimulation of NMDA receptors. Thus, it is hypothesized that **nitric oxide is involved in producing the neurotoxicity and cell disturbances associated with chronic alcohol exposure.** [Alcoholism: Clinical and Experimental Research. Volume 16 Issue, Pages 539 – 541] Published Online: 11 Apr 2006

How do scientists induce consistent, chronic, bowel inflammation in laboratory animals to study bowel inflammation diseases? Chronic inflammation is fueled by nitric oxide. To achieve this, they inject the animals with Enterococcus faecalis and E. faecalis (EF).

Enterococcus faecalis is a Gram-positive commensal bacterium **inhabiting the gastrointestinal tracts of humans** and other mammals. A commensal organism (my note: *commensal* means it needs to live off other organisms), like other species in the genus *Enteroccus*, *E. faecalis* can cause life-threatening infections in humans, especially in the nosocomial (hospital) environment, where the naturally high levels of antibiotic resistance found in *E. faecalis* contribute to its pathogenicity. [Wikipedia]

How does the GI tract of humans become overrun with *E. faecalis*? E. faecalis grows by *fermenting glucose.* Where do you get that glucose? A diet of grains and sugars – *not* the fare best suited for human health (See Chapter 11 *Nature's Medicines*). It doesn't take a rocket scientist to figure out that *not producing those deadly bacteria in the first place* would be the best possible scenario. To do this, consume a diet nearly entirely of pure, fresh, whole, (preferably organic) plant foods. Yet this approach is not at all what you will find from the medical community. In fact, studies continue as we speak to find "the drug" that will treat the inflammation. These drugs come with warnings of internal bleeding, coma, even death. You hear these warnings daily on television drug commercials.

This information should be taken ultra-seriously by *anyone* with any kind of inflammatory disease. Actually, we now know that every disease has an inflammatory component. **Inflammation is the end result and insult to your cells and thus, both causes and accompanies disease.** This means that when a pollutant and then parasite attacks your cells, your cells react by a series of both protective and damage responses which include inflammation. Indeed, anyone wanting to do the best possible thing to begin to reverse and heal their disease, would want to immediately embark upon a diet of *only* pure, fresh, whole, (preferably organic) plant foods. If you are working to get well, your diet should *not* include grains, fiberless sugars (fruits are among the best foods for you and the "sugar" in them is very healthful – by intelligent design, of course!), dairy, alcohol, glutamates, cigarettes, and meats (especially processed). For people with "excess nitric oxide diseases" (like migraines and all painful inflammatory diseases), viral problems, and cancer, no nuts and seeds, either (See Chapter 11 *Nature's Medicines*). So this pure, fresh, whole, (preferably organic) plant food diet actually applies to *everyone* with any kind of disease (and anyone who wants to not come down with a disease).

Chapter 5
ALL THE THINGS GOING ON vs THE "RABBIT"

When you go to the doctor he looks at "all the things going on". He will look at lumps, cuts, lesions, redness and pain, for the purpose of trying to find an antidote in his bag of tricks for any or all of them. It's not uncommon for people over 50 to be taking many different medications all at once. It is also not uncommon for the medications to cause problems that lead to more doctor visits and more drugs to counteract the drugs. When this all fails there's surgery, radiation and even being told "there's nothing more we can do". This is a typical life-time course of medical events for most people.

Not only have I paid for the services of, but I have also worked very closely with "orthodox" as well as "alternative" and "holistic" doctors for over 30 years. Combining this with my own 40+ years of misery with psoriasis, lymphoma, migraines, hip pain, trigeminal neuralgia, herpes outbreaks, multiple sclerosis and more — I have learned truths that I want to leave for my children and anyone else who realizes that only the truth sets you free. In health, that means *not* repeating the same mistakes generation after generation that cause so much pain, suffering, and untimely death. In a nutshell, the *truth* is:

1. With the exception of doctors who brilliantly save life in emergency situations, and repair bodies damaged by accidents, the better part of "medicine" would help mankind more if it ceased and desisted in its current methods, i.e., most drugs, radiation and many surgeries.
2. Even alternative and holistic doctors are befuddled by "all the things going on" in a disease, keeping them from

addressing the underlying cause of disease and supplying natural "antidotes" to assist the body in repairing the damage done *including* detox methods and assisting the body in the production and release of endogenous stem cells.

3. Until we look at disease as well as nutrition and "health" from the Creator's point of view, even people who believe they are in the "health" field will remain confused.

4. The most important truth you're not being told (most doctors ignore this truth, or don't know) is that what's <u>really</u> killing us is *pollutants* first and foremost. It's only after pollutants do their damage that parasites and nutritional deficiencies complicate matters causing *all the things going on.* Even "genetic" diseases are really just damage to genetic material from pollutants in the individual's present and *past* life. This means pollutants that are either passed down from parents and grandparents, or have done genetic damage in ancestors, and the damage itself is passed down.

These four truths led me to the "Rabbit" analogy to help us better understand the truth about what is really causing our epidemic of diseases. I once told this story to a holistic doctor (M.D.) who enthusiastically praised this as a great analogy.

The Rabbit

Imagine a car winding down a country road and a little rabbit runs out in front of the car. The car swerves to miss it and ends up plowing into a very large oak tree. The engine ends up in the front seat, the steering wheel is bent in half, and the front wheel flies off into a ditch. Oil, gas and water are dripping onto the ground beneath the car. There is glass everywhere, a broken antennae, the alarm system goes off and is sounding loudly as the airbags that deployed are now deflating noisily, and a popped tire is also deflating making a hissing sound. Soon an ambulance and highway patrol show up. As the injured occupants are hurried away in the ambulance, the medic's job is established – save the injured peoples' lives if possible.

This leaves the highway patrol to discern *what caused the accident in the first place?* He begins to list the condition of the car, the leaking, the noises, what's broken, where things have gotten out of place and landed, etc., but he still cannot figure out what *caused* the accident. Even subsequent forensic analysis of the vehicle cannot determine the cause. The researchers find that the brakes were working, the steering wheel was working, there was nothing wrong with the engine, etc.

Now imagine the car is your body instead. The highway patrol is your doctor. All too often in medicine, your doctor never discovers that it was one little rabbit that ran across the road and caused a domino effect of other things to happen. **Your doctor (and even you) are so busy gathering up all the "things going on" in your disease you never find the "rabbit".** You do test after test, spend hundreds even thousands of dollars – and you never find the rabbit. And all this, even if you *suspect* a rabbit, because all too often you can no longer see the rabbit. Perhaps he's done his dirty work and has run off (mercury does irreversible damage and then partly leaves the body and partly imbeds deep in your tissues and *bones* where normal tests don't detect it!) Nevertheless, in the case of neurological (as well as other diseases, like cancer) *mercury was the rabbit* . Mercury goes undetected and unsuspected. You go home as much in the dark as before, but now with a list of more tests to do, drugs to take, surgeries to face, and pain to suffer.

What does this all mean? In this particular accident, had there been no rabbit there would have been no accident, and therefore no list of "things going on". Likewise, if we were never to be immunized with vaccines containing toxic metals (like mercury and aluminum), nor have yearly flu shots (mercury), nor have packed mercury into cavities in our teeth (you get the idea - *any* source of toxic metals, like cadmium from smoking or lead from tainted household products or leaded gasoline exhaust, etc.) there would be NO neurological diseases and thus no list of "things going on". Were you or someone you know *born* with a disease (i.e., genetic)? That too was caused by the "rabbit", the pollutant, the mercury, lead, arsenic, cadmium, etc. in your parents' or grandparents' bodies, and the damage passed along to you.

Doctors looking at all the "things going on" notice that there is a rash on the skin, inflammation, a cough, a pain, and begin ordering many tests and then various drugs to put a band-aid over these things going on. Rarely if ever, does the typical doctor seek out the "rabbit", tell you what it is, and then proceed to eradicate it so that your body can *heal*. Our *Creator* didn't design that we would simply "fall apart" for no reason. We have within us a massive and powerful immune system to counteract any "natural" foreign substance that makes its way into our bodies (dirt, dust, undigested protein, virus, etc.). It's the *unnatural* foreign pollutant wrecking havoc, all of which God didn't intend. We are not suppose to carelessly inject, swallow, slather on, breathe, and eat toxic chemicals! Unfortunately, looking for pollutants and their removal as well as natural antidotes to their damage isn't anywhere *near* how doctors perform their duties now or in the past (although they seemed a bit more aware of things a hundred or more years ago – perhaps out of necessity because they had fewer procedures and drugs to offer).

One example of not looking for "the rabbit" at all, is an entire world unable to wrap their mind completely around the fact that a little mercury rabbit can cause 1 in 150 children to get autism today. Children today are given a schedule of some 50+ vaccinations most if not all of which contain thimerosal (mercury) as a "preservative". Compare this to the *single* immunization (small pox) given long ago that corresponded with less than 1 in 2,000 children getting autism. Recently I read that some country removed the mercury and there was still the same rate of autism. First, I question that the mercury has truly been removed – but I also question whether or not these children are still getting mercury in dental work, a diet high in fish, or even lead from imported products (and is this a country where "every" adult smokes?).

It's December, 2008, and mercury is *still* in many vaccines...years after we were told it would be removed. Although even if mercury is removed from vaccines, we still have to avoid fish consumption (how regularly do you eat tuna? salmon?) and never allow amalgams or other toxic metals in your dental work. Dr. Joseph Mercola called a vaccine company and the representative said that even though "thimerosal" has been taken out, *there is still mercury in some vaccines.* She also admitted that flu shots don't even work. Very interesting. Go to: http://articles.mercola.com/sites/articles/archive/2008/11/18/do-flu-shots-work-ask-a-vaccine-manufacturer.aspx or search for "do flu shots work, ask a vaccine manufacturer".

The actress Jenny McCarthy brought her son through autism by realizing that mercury was involved, but then fell short on Larry King Live when he asked her what she thinks caused the autism. Mercury was merely one of many things she lists. In so doing, she illustrates the main point I'm trying to make, and that is, she, like nearly every doctor alive today confuse the underlying cause of something (meaning, "no mercury = no autism") with *all the things going on* (meaning, they wouldn't be going on, if there had been no mercury in the first place). If you didn't know that the wobbling and slowing of your car was due to a flat tire, so you fixed the headlight, would you expect to correct the wobbling and slowing? Of course not.

The truth is, with regard to the 1 in 150 children getting autism from mercury, *many* of the remaining 149 children, are getting childhood Parkinson's, MS, ADHD, migraines, asthma, eczema, psoriasis, diabetes, "allergies", epilepsy and more. In essence, *most* children have "something". This is *not* acceptable! It's not what God intended! Yet it's now so commonplace, that we've come to accept these horrible, disfiguring, painful, expensive, and life-shortening diseases as if they are "normal". A commercial that saddens me is one in which a child coughs while playing on a playground and two moms reach into their purse for anti-allergy medication. A cough is normal! It's the body's way of eliminating phlegm and foreign particles from the lungs! If a child coughs chronically, then find out why – don't cover it up with a chemical!

Another thing that saddens me is when I hear stories like this one. A 12 year old boy, October 2007, died from a Staph infection. I wonder if this poor child had been immunized (mercury) and given antibiotics for earaches and sore throats and such throughout his lifetime – because to *die* so readily from a Staph infection means his immune system was shot. When you hear of children *dying* from the flu or other childhood diseases, it's because their immune system has been so damaged by mercury, lead, pesticides, glutamates and radiation that there just isn't enough immune power there to save them from parasites. As discussed previously, it also means that the overuse of antibiotics has caused resistent strains of bacteria.

So Why Aren't Doctors Looking For The Rabbit?

As I shared previously, I had so many sore throats and other infections throughout junior high and high school I believe I missed more school than went. I was told I had lymphoma in my 20's and started getting horrendous migraines in my 30's. I spent much of each and every day as if in a war zone – combating heavy skin plaques, migraines, easy tendency to sore throats, laryngitis and much more. I was desperately seeking answers. By the age of 40 I had spent thousands upon thousands of dollars of my own money on doctors and I could no longer get medical insurance (they said I "went to the doctor too much"). All that expense – and for absolutely nothing. Indeed, no doctor, no acupuncturist, no nutritionist, no chiropractor could ever find the rabbit. Then I realized that they wouldn't have recognized him had he run across their path! That's not even what they were looking for.

In fact working closely behind the scenes with doctors I learned that for most of them the bottom line to what they did was income to their practice. I actually sat in on medical staff office meetings where the discussions were of the type and quality of insurance various patients had – not how the doctors could help specific patients! Even though a close friend of the doctors I worked for I was surprised to find that never was any extra effort made on their part to help me with my own health issues.

There are hundreds of disease "names"...but really only a few common causes. Whenever you hear of anyone with a disease, the first thing that *should* come to your mind is, "Which pollutant(s)? *Then* which parasite(s)? Until you only seek answers to those questions, you'll wander from doctor to doctor, test to test, getting nowhere. At the same time you have to ask, "Are there any deficiencies complicating matters and making me even more susceptible?" And what you should *never* buy into again is when doctors and scientists try to dismiss something as being "genetic" as if you have absolutely no control over anything. Genetic diseases exist, no denying that, but what that really means is that the person's genes were damaged or mutated <u>by a pollutant</u>! If you're born with it, then it happened in the womb or was passed on from a mutated gene from a parent. If it happens after you're born, then a gene mutated as you grew outside the womb. We study genetic diseases backwards. The *first* thing we need to do is *stop* the damage in the first place. That means getting *rid* completely of the mercury, the lead, the asbestos, the cadmium, the phthalates (plastics), etc. How much sense does it make to you, that if your ship is sinking, you keep bailing out the water, but don't plug up the hole?

When We Need Doctors

We need doctors when we get in a car accident and need to be sewn back together. We *don't* need doctors to give us medications for every ailment without knowing what causes the ailment. Take restless leg syndrome. RLS is nasty, by the way, nothing to make jokes about – and is yet another neurological disease. But the answer is to *stop eating excitotoxins (see section on glutamates) and stop injecting yourself with mercury.* You don't heal by adding insult to injury with a toxic drug. RLS has also been associated with migraines [see: Rhode A et al. Comorbidity of migraine and restless legs syndrome-a case-control study. *Cephalgia.* 2007 Sep 210]. The reason migraines and RLS are related is that restless leg syndrome is a neurological firestorm in the legs, just as a migraine is a neurological firestorm in the brain. Restless leg syndrome is worse at night, especially after a meal that either supplies or stimulates free glutamates. We've all seen the commercials about how you can use a medication with possible "fatal" side effects for your restless legs, dry eyes or arthritis. They list blood clots, heart attack, even cancer, as "side effects". I cannot believe anyone would run to get a prescription!

The next time you go to a doctor, make sure you know why you're going. I go to confirm a diagnosis. I go prepared with as much information as I can gather. I don't go to get a prescription or injection. As for me, I'll only go now to have something sewn back on or in a coma, on a stretcher.

Chapter 6
DENTAL WORK – THE ROOTS OF DISEASE

How Many Teeth Do You Have?

In December of 2007 I was the proud owner of 28 teeth. They were all white and so beautiful – not typical in the mouth of your average 54 year old. So "beautiful" were they, in fact, that a doctor, looking down my throat exclaimed, "my compliments to your dentist!" Then, in February of 2008 I did a *radical* thing (definition: **radical** *adv* to get to the root cause). I had my three root canals taken *out.* The first was of necessity – the crown had popped off while flossing, and underneath was bloody and infected. That root canal had been done "biologically", that is, using laser and a "natural" material called biocalyx, but it rotted anyway! When that crown popped off, what was underneath was absolutely disgusting. This incident told me the other two root canals would go the same route – but that in the meantime, diseased roots were likely *contributing* to my diseases and pain! And I was in a lot of pain.

This was no easy thing to do, emotionally – *remove* what appeared on the outside at least, to be *"perfectly good"* teeth? What a frightening thought! Will I look the same, can I eat my salads? I'm a professional singer….will that end? I felt I had no choice, but it also hasn't been an easy road finding the right dentist. The few that claim to do it according to the work of Dr. Price (see books listed below) seem to walk the fence between doing it right and "big business".

I found a dentist an hour away, and chose her over flying to another state. Long story very short - when I had my root canals out the dentist removed five perfectly good crowns (non-metal) and replaced them with non-metal crowns. X-rays show that the new crowns aren't as good as the old ones were! I'm having trouble with those teeth now. I'm sharing this hoping you'll investigate your local dentists very carefully long before you need them. You've got to find the best "biological" dentist you can.

"Your overall health is at stake...not the life of a single, motley tooth". Hal Huggins

I began reading all the books I could get on the subject:

1. Dr. Hal Huggins "Uninformed Consent" and "It's All In Your Head",
2. Dr. Mark A. Breiner's "Whole Body Dentistry"
3. Dr. George Meinig's "Root Canal Cover-Up" *based upon the work of Dr. Weston Price*
4. Dr. Robert Kulacz' "The Root's of Disease, Connecting Dentistry & Medicine", and
5. Dr. Martin Fischer's "Death and Dentistry".

I learned that even crowns aren't good because bacteria grows underneath. These too, can change in the anaerobic environment and create toxins that contribute to disease. Well, I'm not ready to extract *all* my teeth (of the 25 teeth left, 8 are crowns). Thankfully crowns aren't nearly as bad as root canals. In fact, if you suspect there is some decay under a crown, you can sometimes have the crown removed, the decay cleaned up a bit, and the crown replaced.

In my search for a good biological dentist, before finding the one who pulled my root canals, I went to a gentleman who takes people down into Mexico for their dentistry. There are many who claim to practice biologically down there. He told me this:

I obtain my dental products from Germany. Germany has basically banned dental procedures including mercury, root canals, and crowns because they know the toxic results to be the most prevalent contributor to the world's epidemic of diseases. No, the government doesn't come right out and say "dentistry is banned" – yet. Apparently they've given all dentists a certain number of years to become maxillofacial surgeons before issuing an outright ban on "orthodox" dental practices. They plan in the future to not insure or treat anyone who comes to, say, an emergency room having a stroke...if they have mercury fillings, root canals, etc. He said that Germany currently makes the finest dental prosthetics, like dentures and partials. Go to: http://www.zeromercury.org/press/250507_Mercury%20_Dental_PR.pdf where you'll learn that Sweden, Denmark and Norway are banning mercury.

Then I found this:

The Townsend Letter, a well-known journal for holistic medicine practitioners, announced recently (in 2008) that **mercury** has been **banned** from all dental fillings in Norway. From the beginning of this year dentists in Norway have to start using safer alternatives. The ban goes further than amalgam fillings, covering many other products; including measuring instruments such as thermometers and sphygmomanometers for measuring blood pressure.

Well, it was a pretty horrific experience, having those three teeth pulled all at once. I suffered a lot of pain and healing time. But the really good news is that after taking out the three root canals, after 20 years of horrific suffering, *I no longer have 10+ debilitating migraines.* The "headaches" I continue to get are only a 2-3 on the 1-10 scale, whereas the migraines had been 10+ every single time, and accompanied by severe nausea. I used to have to go to bed for 1-3 days and often begged God to just take me. Now I take an Excedrin and lots of ginger, and can function all day. I will continue now armed with truth and do what is needed as the need arises, like *pull* a diseased tooth rather than do a root canal. So why did taking out those root canals have such a profound effect?

Chronic Infections From Your Root Canals & Other Sources

Why are root canals the worst dental contributors to disease bodywide? The reason is because normally you *know* when you have an infection. But because a root canal, by definition is the removal of the nerve from the root, you can have a raging infection and not know it. The nerve is gone, so you feel nothing. That you can't feel any pain is the first reason a chronic infection from root canals is among the most dangerous. Remember, when my crown popped off the root canaled tooth, underneath was black and bloody. I hadn't felt any pain at all, not at the site of the tooth, that is.

The second reason root canals are the most dangerous, is because the bacteria produces deadly toxins in the anaerobic environment of the root tubules. This bacteria and its toxins cannot be reached by your immune system, nor by oxygen, while in those tubules. The toxins leave the tubules and travel throughout the body setting up infections elsewhere. The close proximity of the teeth to the brain is one reason the bacteria travels readily up into the brain.

"...Remember, there are good bacteria and there are even more pathogenic, or disease-causing bacteria...sometimes "good" bacteria can *become* "bad" bacteria. Just like *Clostridium botulinum,* the species of bacteria that produces the extremely potent toxin associated with botulism, many bacteria normally found in the mouth are virtually harmless to the body until their oxygen supply is taken away. Once this occurs, the lack of oxygen changes the metabolism of the bacteria, and enormously toxic bacterial metabolic by-products are produced: harmless bacteria of the mouth will produce similarly potent toxins when trapped in the oxygen-starved environment of the dentin tubules of a root canal treated tooth." [Robert Kulacz DDS, *The Roots of Disease,* Connecting Dentistry & Medicine 2002]

Some scientists might quibble over the potential for bacteria to "become" bad bacteria. *Sherris Medical Microbiology* says that bacteria do, indeed, mutate, and they do so rapidly. I have to believe that actual evidence supports this. Below, we see that over 150 strains of bacteria have been identified within or surrounding a dead or dying tooth, and all but five are anaerobic. If there wasn't a mutation, from where then, did the anaerobic bacteria come?

> Over 150 different bacterial strains have been identified at the apex or within the pulp chamber of dead or dying teeth. All but five are classified as anaerobic. These bacteria produce waste products known as toxins. No matter which direction the toxins go, they will be introduced to the innermost portions of the host's body. [Hal A. Huggins DDS, MS from **Uninformed Consent** The Hidden Dangers In Dental Care.]

One study was performed to determine whether chronic dental infections (and other types of infections) are a risk factor for cerebrovascular ischemia. Cerebrovascular ischemia stimulates nitric oxide production, and excess nitric oxygen in individuals with mercury damage to the glutamatergic system, leads to migraine and stroke.

> *Conclusion:* Recurrent or chronic bronchial infection and poor dental status, mainly resulting from **chronic dental infection**, may be associated with an **increased risk for cerebrovascular ischemia.** [*Stroke.* 1997;28:1724-1729]

It's Not Just Root Canals, Though

Any dental procedure that introduces a toxic substance (like mercury or nickel), or creates an environment in which bacteria can thrive, is what contributes to diseases bodywide (see focal infection, below). One such situation is when teeth are removed without completing the job. Here's what Dr. Hal Huggins says in his book:

> When teeth are removed, the **periodontal ligament** (a membrane that atttaches the tooth to the bone) is usually left in the socket. I now compare this membrane to the afterbirth that is delivered after a baby is born. If the afterbirth is left in, the mother will probably die. When the periodontal ligament is left in, the patient does not die, but neither does the socket area completely heal. I have found that the top of the socket seals over with two or three millimeters of bone; under that, a hole remains. This bony hole is usually lined with *chronic inflammatory lymphocyctes*, which are the cells of autoimmune disease. [Hal Huggins DDS, *It's All In Your Head – The Link Between Mercury Amalgams and Illness* 1993.]

Unfortunately (or fortunately, depending upon how you look at it) I experienced this firsthand, and long before I'd read about it in Dr. Huggin's book. When I had that very first infected root canal removed, it was done by an "orthodox" dentist who merely pulled it out, gave me gauze to bite on and sent me home. That socket got terribly infected, and I suffered horrifically until I found the dentist who knew to pull the ligament and clean out the socket. Furthermore, an infection in the teeth and roots doesn't stay in one place, but travels throughout the body. This is called a "focal infection".

Focal Infection

If you have any chronic pain, like in your hip, your shoulder, your knee, *migraines* – anything, and anywhere – and you have no clearcut explanation for that chronic pain, consider the following: Dr. Meinig, in *Root Canal Coverup* wrote that people who have infections in their mouth, especially from decaying root canals (but also under crowns) will have "focal infections" throughout the body. Of course we've been discussing infections traveling from the mouth and going throughout the body, and settling in some far off area, and here now we have a name for the phenomenon, i.e., **focal infections.**

Bacteria in an infected tooth can mutate, even becoming anerobic bacteria that produce deadly toxins which travel throughout the body causing damage and chronic pain. The definition of a focal infection is a bacterial infection that is limited to one place in the body (like in a root canaled tooth, or under a crown), but causes symptoms somewhere else in the body. This is *not* just a theory. Dr. Meinig's book is based upon the 25 years of scientific studies by Dr. Weston A. Price. Dr. Price would take root canaled teeth out of people who had a disease like arthritis, implant the tooth under the skin of a rabbit, and the rabbit would develop the very same disease the person had! He did this over and over again, and the rabbit never failed to develop the exact same disease as the person with the infected tooth had.

While dentists and doctors alike are *still* trying to ignore the truth of focal infections, Dr. Thomas Rau, director of a medical clinic in Switzerland will tell he estimates that 90% of all infections that he has observed in his patients are caused by bacteria from dental infections. Please do not take this lightly. Notice for yourself how often a person with a mouthful of root canals and crowns ends up with the worst diseases, and the folks living into their 90's or even over 100 without disabling neurological diseases or cancer, either have had all their teeth removed or still have all their teeth but very little to no dental work! I've been connecting these two (good health with good or no teeth, in other words, a mouth *without* mercury or infection) for years! In fact, I now believe the infection in holes created in my jaw from incomplete removal of my wisdom teeth is what contributed most to my migraines. Prior to having the three root canals removed, the dentist pointed to an x-ray of the area of my wisdom teeth and said, "There…that's the ligament they left in."

So, again, I have proven the focal infection theory to not be a theory at all. Removal of three root canals along with cleaning up "debris" of previously removed teeth (removing the periodontal ligament and cavitations – those are the name for the unhealed holes created from teeth removal) caused a history of horrific migraines from 10+ for 3 days with nausea, vomiting, and frequent trips to the emergency room and many, many thousands of out-of-pocket dollars to doctors and ERs - to reduce down to no greater than 2-3 in severity, no more nausea, and migraines that are now easily handled by OTC medications. In addition many other infections throughout the body became less frequent, less severe and some even disappeared. To top it off, when some of my teeth began to rot under crowns, some of my focal infections began to slowly return – hip pain in particular.

Simply stated, the **focal infection theory** takes the position that infected teeth, tonsils, tonsil tags, sinuses and such areas of infection contain bacteria which can travel to another gland, organ or tissue and set up a new infection site. Dr. Weston Price was not the only doctor carrying out research on this subject. …what makes these bacteria so dangerous is their ability to become polymorphic; that is, to mutate, adapt, change, become smaller, anaerobic, more virulent and more toxic. [2007 Sung Lee, and George Meinig D.D.S]

That dental infections can cause much disease, even death is not new. In fact, in a documentary, Secrets of Egypt's Lost Queen, played on The Discovery Channel, July 17, 2008 we learned of Hatshepsut, a female, born in about 1500 BC. She was the beautiful daughter of Tuthmosis I (her father). Upon the pharaoh's death his son by another wife, Tuthmosis II, in turn became pharaoh. Hatshepsut then married Tuthmosis II ("incest" was allowed in Egyptian royal families). When Hatshepsut's husband died in about 1479BC, his son by a harem girl, Tuthmosis III, was in line to be pharaoh but was only a young boy. So Hatshepsut took the throne and held onto it until about 1458 BC, when she died and Tuthmosis III (now grown into a man) belatedly claimed it. There has been speculation how she died all these years (she was only 42 if you've done the math). Many have speculated that Tuthmosis III hated her and killed her. But recent discoveries in her tomb revealed that she died of an **abscessed molar!**

Are You "Dying" From Infections In Your Root Canals and Under Your Crowns?

As I said, after taking out my three root canals, and cleaning up cavitations, etc., my migraines virtually disappeared. At this writing it's been over a year now, and I've still not had a migraine with nausea or vomiting. Neither have I had a migraine that sent me to bed covering my head and eyes with ice for days at a time, and suffering so badly I prayed for God to just take me. Yet for some 20 years, these would happen up to three times per month!

However, I still have some crowns, and they are beginning to develop infections under them (the infection can be felt, smelled and even tasted when you are aware). A chronic hip pain that left for many months has returned though not as often nor as bad. I'm looking at needing to have these decaying teeth out, and getting a "partial" to replace the teeth I will lose. I can assure you, I will welcome being completely out of pain again – and hopefully for the rest of my life. I *don't* welcome the prospect of pulling more teeth. But I wonder just how many people have a mouthful of crowns and implants and their health gets worse and worse every day. They don't even connect the two! Yet we all know such people. Their smile may even look good – amazing in fact, that an 85 year old, say, would have a mouthful of what on the surface appears to be beautiful white teeth. Unless they are the teeth God gave them, I can assure you, under each crown is an infection that is causing "focal infections" throughout their body. This can and *does* lead to everything from arthritis to diabetes, to heart disease or cancer. A personal observation of mine has been that nearly every person I've met with a mouthful of crowns has severe and chronic halitosis – caused by bacteria of course.

You Will Have To Remind Yourself Why You Took Such Radical Steps

As I sit here, currently with 25 of the 28 teeth I had only 10 months ago, I am writing a "note to self" to remind myself that taking out mercury, root canals and even crowns that are decaying underneath isn't optional – it's a must. I know how "quickly we forget" when pain is gone. I am well aware that underneath the eight or so crowns I still have, there is brown/black and decay, which is producing bacteria that is producing toxins. I'm personally not ready at this very moment to act preemptively and pull out all my crowns (nor do I believe I need to), but I know that as needed, decayed crowned teeth must go, cavitations must never be allowed (read the recommended books), any mercury left must be cleaned up, no root tips anywhere. I can still have beautiful white teeth, they'll just have to be manufactured in a lab.

I'm taking the best care I can of the teeth I have left by not eating sugar, flossing after I eat, and brushing properly. I swish my mouth with hydrogen peroxide as well to lessen the bacteria population (I believe it's a perfectly natural method to do this, and it has the added benefit of whitening the teeth!)

You're Going To Encounter Opposition

I can't tell you how many times I told a "laser" dentist I was going to because I couldn't find a better dentist: "I don't do root canals". He would tell me he's going to *convince* me that root canals are fine. And this, after I told him of the expense and pain I went through *removing* three root canals – one of which had been done "holistically" (exactly like he does them), yet *rotted!* But that's not all! I even told him of my 20 year history with horrific migraines, virtually *gone* immediately after removing the root canals. And this, after 20 years of trying every therapy, every herb, every medicine to little avail. But how could I, sitting in the dentist's chair, in just a minute or two, explain over 20 years of suffering (migraines), to where he would understand? The answer of course is that I couldn't.

I resorted to giving that dentist reading materials. I gave him Dr. Meinig's "Root Canal Coverup". But I don't expect his stance to change because he's obviously following the "business model" of dentistry, and not the "truth model". I actually appreciate a dentist's desire to cash in on his years of education. Over the years that I've worked for various doctors I've done their bookkeeping, both business and personal. I also did their medical billing, their medical assisting, and their medical office management. So I can thoroughly appreciate that they have expensive training and expensive equipment not to mention an office, employees and a family to support. They *must* earn money. This very dentist confessed that doing root canals and crowns is the way to make that money (although he was referring to the other dentist who sold me unnecessary crowns).

He also told me he didn't have much time to read. This is tragic, too, because when I asked him if he knew of Dr. Weston Price's 1,174 pages of studies based upon 25 years of work by 60 scientists showing how damaging root canals are to the immune system and health, he said he'd *never heard of these studies.* With what I know now, that actually makes me feel like I've been punched in the stomach. *Every* practicing dentist should know about Dr. Price's 25 years of research! How can *anything* be done right for their patients when the truths Dr. Weston found aren't known?

Even with the best dentists I've known (and I've been to plenty) not only are they all on the "business model" path, but all have turned into dental "car mechanics". Indeed, the way in which they practice dentistry bears little distinction from working on a car – with one main exception. That is, mechanics remove the old spark plugs and put in new ones. They flush out the engine. They put air in the tires. With cars they never have to worry that a flat tire, say, is "infecting" the radiator. *But that's not the way it is in dentistry.* I've often thought if I could only capture my dentist's attention long enough, and if I believed he really cared, I'd tell him that human beings are not like cars. The tooth upon which a root canal is performed is not a lone entity, and does, indeed, have an effect on the rest of the body. That tooth, that root, that blood supply, those nerves…they're all *attached to the rest of my body.* When the root, denied of oxygen from a healthy blood and nerve supply begins to harbor dangerous anaerobic bacteria, those bacteria *travel* through the body's systems, to the central nervous system, the brain…indeed, the entire body. To date, I've made zero headway trying to explain this to any "orthodox", "holistic" *or* "laser" dentist. There are only a handful of dentists in this entire country that truly "get it". These are the ones that practice dentistry according to the 25 years of research of Weston Price DDS.

Prevention

1. First, *prevent* tooth decay by making sure you get enough calcium and other minerals internally, and by keeping your mouth the proper pH by not consuming starches/sugars (except 100% natural as in fruits or vegetables).
2. Brush with a *non-fluouride* toothpaste as often as you need to *keep* your teeth free of food adhering to them. (Try JASON paste with tea tree oil, its wonderful)
3. *Floss* often, even after every meal! An excellent natural floss also has tea tree oil in it.
4. Scrape off any *plaque* you see – daily. You can purchase dental tools at most pharmacies that do this.
5. Whiten teeth and get rid of bacteria in the mouth by swishing with *hydrogen peroxide*. Just 15-30 seconds once or twice daily is all that is needed – and you have the added bonus of whitening your teeth naturally.

DENTAL MUSTS:

a) YES to biocompatible material (composite or white) fillings. I've heard that "Diamond" is one of the best.

b) YES to Diamond or LAVA (cubic zirconium) crowns (but only when a filling can absolutely no longer be used....hold out for the filling as long as you can!) or any completely metal-free, non-toxic materials as may come along in the future

c) YES to pulling a root damaged tooth but only by a dentist that knows how to clean out the periodontal ligament and cavitations. Ask if they do according to the work of Dr. Weston Price. Ask if they even know who Dr. Weston Price is! (You can buy them Dr. Kulacz' and Meinig's books – see "Recommended Reading" - to educate them if necessary)

d) **YES** to Valplast partials or any made of biocompatible materials

e) **YES** to digital x-rays only, *and* as few x-rays as possible

f) **NO** to mercury

g) **NO** to any metal at all even "high noble" or whatever else they want to call it

h) **NO** to root canals

Chapter 7
PSORIASIS

After reading this you should understand that in psoriasis there is widespread **damage by mercury** to the **intestinal barrier**, **kidneys**, **immune system**, **glutathione** system of detoxification, coupled with the resultant **overgrowth of Candida**, (which ironically has an affinity for mercury). The *Candida* leads to **"leaky gut"** where macroparticles of undigested foods as well as "endotoxins" from the *Candida,* and pollutants (like pesticides, antibiotics, food additives and more) go freely into the bloodstream where a damaged and now overwhelmed immune system (of which glutathione is an important player) does its best to protect you from the toxins. The end result is the skin acting as an extraordinary means of elimination (the exudation of psoriasis), which causes the inflammation (the skin wasn't meant to deal with such a heavy load). There are many other things "going on", but the entire process ending in psoriasis was *caused* by mercury.

The *Cause* Of Psoriasis

The cause of psoriasis is mercury, because no mercury = no psoriasis. In psoriasis the lining of the gut has been damaged (both by mercury and by candida because of mercury's damage to the immune system) and now various undigested food substances, antibiotics, pesticides, toxins produced by the candida (called antigens i.e., *foreign substances*) are crossing the damaged barrier, getting into the bloodstream and setting up all the "things going on" that end in exudation and inflammation of the skin - *psoriasis*. Many classify psoriasis and other skin disorders as "allergic disorders" in that foreign substances in the bloodstream set up a cascade of events leading to the outward appearance of skin redness, exudations, rashes, etc.

The underlying denominators and treatment targets in allergic disorders may be outlined as **aberrant barrier functions of the skin epithelium and gut mucosa** and dysregulation of the immune response to ubiquitous environmental antigens. [*J Clin Gastroenterol* 2008 Jul;42 Suppl 2:S91-6.]

Why I Don't Eat Non-Fat Frozen Yogurt Anymore

Once the body has been damaged by mercury, those foods and substances that you may have "handled" for many years, may now become toxic. Carrageenan is just one of those substances. In fact, carrageenan is just one of the thousands of reasons (thousands of possible food additives, that is) why you should eat only pure, whole, fresh, (preferably organic) plant foods. Just considering carrageenan as one of the many thousands of food additives may give you a hint as to how potentially dangerous all others can be as well.

But people have reached a point of "oblivion" when it comes to food additives. To be sure, we are so used to seeing foreign nomenclature on the list of "ingredients" in such products as "Hot Pockets" or Campbell's soup that we've resigned ourselves to trust the food manufacturer. But don't! Even when/if they boast "no MSG" *read the label!*

Carrageenan is a stabilizer, texturizer, thickener, and gelling agent in the food and pharmaceutical industries. Some call it a "vaseline-like" substance. You will find it mostly in "creamy" foods like those soft-serve frozen yogurts, for example. But Carrageenan has an evil side:

> Multiple studies in animal models have shown that the commonly used food additive **carrageenan** (CGN) induces inflammation and intestinal neoplasia. Human colonic epithelial cells that were exposed to CGN for 1-8 d, we found increased cell death, reduced cell proliferation, and cell cycle arrest compared with unexposed control cells. CGN exposure may have **a role in development of human intestinal pathology.** [*J Nutr* 2008 Mar;138(3):469-75.]

One of the things going on in psoriasis is *intestinal pathology.* **Carrageenan causes intestinal inflammation and damage.**

It All Started With A Mouthful Of Amalgams

I started out as a normal, healthy child! When I was young I had the usual sore throats and "childhood" diseases. Other than that, I was healthy and normal. No allergies, no skin diseases, no asthma, no diabetes, no attention deficit disorder - nothing. In fact, not too long ago my mother announced at a family get-together where we were all discussing our childhood health histories, that she thought I'd had a very "normal childhood" - nothing out of the ordinary. We were a family of nine who rarely went to the doctor (knowing what I know now...*thank God* for that!) I <u>didn't</u> have the 50+ immunizations that children are given today (corresponding with approximately 1 in 150 children now with autism – and others in the remaining 149 who get epilepsy, ADD, ADHD, asthma, allergies, diabetes, cancer and more from the mercury).

I was healthy that is, until the age of 11. It was somewhere in my 11th year that I remember having an abscess in a back molar. I had gone to the dentist and after an examination he exclaimed: "You have eight cavities!" As I said, we didn't go to doctors or dentists but once or twice in our entire childhood. Well, I returned to the dentist for "fillings" and within a week or two I had a mouthful of shiny "silver" fillings. But what I didn't know then, and know all too well now, is those "silver" fillings were composed *not* just of silver, but contain over 50% of a highly toxic metal - mercury. I suppose I wouldn't have understood what that meant anyway as we were using "mercurochrome" as an antiseptic at the time. Mercurochrome was subsequently banned (1998) by the FDA as not safe.

A patient suffering from long-standing pustular **psoriasis** of the palms was treated for 3 weeks with a **mercury-containing drug**. Exacerbation into generalized pustular psoriasis developed. Mercury levels in blood and urine were increased. After withdrawal of the mercury preparation, therapy with DMPA (2,3-Dimercapto-1-propane-sulfonic acid), a mercury antidote was initiated, together with short-term treatment with aromatic retinoids and PUVA. Within a few days mercury levels decreased significantly and the skin lesions practically disappeared. [Hautarzt. 1994 Oct;45(10):708-10.]

Well, after having those eight *mercury* fillings placed, it was only a matter of months when I broke out all over my body with psoriasis [also age 11]. Why?

The reason is that mercury does massive damage to the immune and elimination systems. Consequently, since the age of 11, I have suffered with and continue to fight psoriasis, but I've also suffered from other indications of an injured immune system, and that is, frequent "cold sores", trigeminal neuralgia, tonsillitis, ulcers, hip pain, shingles, migraines, lymphoma, and multiple sclerosis – all from widespread cellular and immune system damage.

A direct mechanism involving **mercury's inhibition of cellular enzymatic processes by binding with the hydroxyl radical(SH) in amino acids appears to be a major part of the connection to allergic/immune reactive conditions** such as autism, schizophrenia, lupus, eczema and **psoriasis**, scleroderma, and allergies. Immune reactivity to mercury has been documented by immune reactivity tests to be a major factor in many of the autoimmune conditions...

[From Shirley's Wellness Café]

Only About The Second Time I Ever Went To A Doctor

After seeing I was covered from head to toe with redness and thick scales, my mother took me to a pediatrician to discern what the problem was. The doctor recognized it right away as psoriasis and suggested I take some type of "horse pill" that I recall having a strong "rotten egg" smell. The doctor had apparently given me a sulfonamide drug, which were among the first antibiotics. He thought my psoriasis was bacterial? Sulfonamides are often not well tolerated. Luckily for me I couldn't swallow pills, and this one was a whopper.

I learned, instead, to soak in the tub and rub off the scales. As a teen with so many other battles to fight in daily life, this battle was enormous, and unfair. Then my mother came home with "Tegrin", which I began to put on the psoriasis, and it would soften the thick, nasty scales so I could rub them off much easier. It smelled awful, and made me even more reclusive. Today I use a non-oily, odor-free gel with salicylic acid (the natural substance in aspirin) called "Dermarest", a *medicated skin treatment*. Dermarest is freely available in most pharmacies. I put it all over my scalp, and can leave it on all day, or just an hour before showering. It works beautifully to soften scaling for easier removal during showering, and washes off well. To the contrary, regular lotions I'd tried had various types of waxes in them that would not wash off well at all.

Unfortunately Tegrin contains "coal tar", which is not desirable. It's action is supposed to slow the scaling process, and while Tegrin never did that for me, a topical I currently use, called "Exorex", does it very well. Exorex also contains coal tar, so I use tiny amounts of it where my psoriasis is visible. It works better than anything I've ever used, but like all chemicals, should be used sparingly, or not at all if you don't feel the need. Currently my psoriasis is mild from the proper diet and use of various immune-enhancing supplements, so I am able to use as little of the topical as possible. You'll find sources of Exorex on the internet.

Indeed, if you have psoriasis, your doctor will prescribe creams and salves and dangerous "antiinflammatory" medicines. He won't tell you, because he doesn't know, that psoriasis is a defect along your immune and elimination system – a defect in your ability to destroy and eliminate antigens (foreign materials) in the gut, the body, the bloodstream. When there is a defect in the normal eliminatory processes, then the skin (a major eliminatory organ) will take up some of the slack. This is the case in "exudative" skin diseases like psoriasis. The inflammation is part and parcel of the irritation put upon the skin to do far more than it was designed to do.

Again, the *cause* of psoriasis is mercury damage to the immune and eliminatory systems of the body. The kidneys, for example, are perhaps our most important eliminatory organ, the blood filters through the kidneys, and wastes are removed. Mercury is known to damage the kidneys.

> Reactive oxygen species are implicated as mediators of tissue damage in the **acute renal failure** induced by inorganic **mercury**. [*Food Chem Toxicol.* 2008 Jan;46(1):212-9.]

Even holistic doctors go to great pains to list all the "things going on" like complicated-sounding cGMP and cAMP (compounds that proliferate and mature your cells) being somehow "awry" in psoriatics. You'll likely hear, "it's genetic", which is what some doctors or scientists say when they haven't got a clue. The truth is that "genetic" means that the genes of the person (or their parents, or grandparents) were damaged/mutated. How were they damaged/mutated? By pollutants, like mercury, of course!

Mercury exerts a variety of toxic effects in the body. Lipid peroxidation, DNA damage and **depletion of reduced glutathione** by Hg(II) suggest an oxidative stress-like mechanism for Hg(II) toxicity. [Basic & Clinical Pharmacology & Toxicology, Volume 93, Number 6, December 2003 , pp. 290-296(7)]

What Is Glutathione?

Glutathione is a small protein composed of three amino acids: cysteine, glutamic acid and glycine. After mercury damages the glutamatergic system, a deficiency in the internal production of glutathione can easily occur both because glutathione works to detoxify the mercury, and also because a body damaged by mercury will have more difficulty producing glutathione.

In a group of 30 people with psoriasis, most were found selenium deficient. They also showed **low levels of a key protein in the blood called "glutathione."** The body uses this protein to make a key antioxidant enzyme called "glutathione peroxidase." Even more suggestive was the finding that people with the most severe psoriasis had the lowest levels of glutathione peroxidase. [Pol Merkuriusz Lek. May1999;6(35):263-5.]

Glutathione is one of the most important compounds in the body involved in detoxification. Glutathione binds to toxins such as heavy metals, solvents, pesticides, medications (like Tylenol) preventing them, literally, from killing you by breaking them down and then escorting them out of your body via urine or bile. Your body manufacturers glutathione, or you intake glutathione when you consume pure, whole, fresh fruits and vegetables, for example. Unfortunately, an attempt to supplement glutathione can be ineffective, damaging, or even painful (migraines, for example) in many people with damaged glutamatergic systems, because it breaks down into its component parts and becomes a source of free glutamates (see Chapter 8 *Migraines*).

Many things "go on" in psoriasis. But they are *still* just "all the things going on." *Mercury* causes the initial damage within the body that ends in the inflammation and exudation of psoriasis. This exudation and inflammation of the skin is what doctors usually treat. At my worst, I had over 80% body coverage of very thick, ugly plaques that would crack and bleed and they completely covered my scalp. It was a miserable childhood, miserable teenage years, and it is still a miserable challenge to combat as an adult. Had I not been "injected" with mercury in the form of amalgams I would *not* have gotten psoriasis!

You Absorb Mercury From The Amalgams In Your Teeth

Your teeth are living, breathing parts of your body, and what you place into them goes into the blood for bodywide distribution. Mercury vapors also escape when you chew. Mercury disables the immune system because it destroys DNA and the cell's mitochondria (energy) - *irreparably*.

The more mercury from immunizations and amalgams—the more you destroy the body's DNA, mitochondria and immune system, creating a scenario for the worse disease potential.

As shown above, mercury also damages the kidneys which are the body's blood filter, cleansing the blood of debris, toxins and wastes. Mercury has an affinity for the brain. Those who say it quickly leaves the body are grossly in error. They only *think* the mercury left. In reality, mercury imbeds itself deep in bone, brain and other tissues where normal urine or blood tests don't find it.

In fact, studies on lab animals have been done to see if calcitonin has any effect on keeping mercury or lead from being taken up by the bones. Calcitonin is a hormone produced by the thyroid gland that lowers the levels of calcium and phosphate in the blood and promotes the formation of bone. When lab animals are given calcitonin:

> Calcitonin dramatically reduced the initial **uptake of lead and mercury by bone.** [Norimatsu, H & Talmage, RV Influence of calcitonin on the initial uptake of lead and mercury by bone, *Proc. Soc. Exp. Biol. Med.* ; Vol/Issue: 161:1]

These particular researchers say they don't know *why* the calcitonin kept the lead and mercury from imbedding into the bone. But what we can learn from this in general, is that when everything is working properly in the human body, for example, you have enough of an essential mineral (like calcium), the body can protect you from toxic elements, like lead or mercury. This is because there are "sites" on cells that hold a calcium atom, and if a calcium atom isn't there (you are deficient) a heavy metal can slip right in and fill that empty space.

In fact, if you hear a siren go off and learn that a nearby nuclear plant has exploded, you'll want to make sure you immediately take extra iodine to protect you from radioactive fallout. The iodine protects your thyroid by preventing the radioactive fallout material from occupying sites meant for iodine.

Well, I didn't connect mercury with psoriasis for many years, in fact, not for about 40 more years. Unfortunately, the years that followed my 11th were filled with headaches, "hives", sore throats, eye sties, herpes outbreaks and more – all of which are an indication of immune and elimination systems not working. I found that when I eliminated pollutants to the best of my ability, ate right and boosted my immune system with herbs, zinc, vitamin C and other supplements, I would go from thick plaques to thinner; from 80% body coverage to 5%, etc. But psoriasis is like type I diabetes in that mercury has done *devastating damage* that can persist for a lifetime. Someday, stem cells will be what reverses the damage, and better still, the complete ban of mercury will mean no more psoriasis in the first place!

There will be some wise-guys that will surface, trying to tell you that of the two different forms of mercury, ethylmercury (inorganic) and methylmercury (organic) one is safe and the other is not. They'll say that amalgams are "ethyl", and the mercury is harmless, doesn't go to the brain, or damage anything. As usual, this has proven to be hogwash. Both "ethyl" and "methyl" are lethal (ultimately). Pun intended. One very wise Dr. Haley said:

"...there is **no safe level of mercury**, and no one has actually shown that there is a safe level. I would say mercury is a very toxic substance..." Dr Lars Friberg, 1920-2006, Former Chief Adviser to the World Health Organization on Mercury safety.

The scientific studies back this professor up as well. Studies with baby monkeys showed that when the type of mercury that is in vaccines and amalgams is injected into these babies, it *does, indeed, head straight* for the brain! This is important, because even today scientists and doctors still pose the "organic" vs. "inorganic" argument as if one type of mercury is perfectly safe. Not so!

We compared the systemic disposition and brain distribution of total and inorganic mercury in infant monkeys after thimerosal (ethylmercury) exposure with those exposed to MeHg (methylmercury). **A higher percentage of the total Hg in the brain was in the form of inorganic Hg for the thimerosal-exposed monkeys (34% vs. 7%)**. The results indicate that MeHg is not a suitable reference for risk assessment from exposure to thimerosal-derived Hg. Knowledge of the toxicokinetics and developmental toxicity of thimerosal is needed to afford a meaningful assessment of the developmental effects of thimerosal-containing vaccines. [Thomas M. Burbacher et al. Comparison of Blood and Brain Mercury Levels in Infant Monkeys Exposed to Methylmercury or Vaccines Containing Thimerosal *Environ Health Perspect* 113: 1015-1021 (2005)]

A "fact sheet" for healthcare professionals on the safe handling of mercury (or avoidance of mercury) also says this:

Elemental or inorganic forms can be transformed into organic (especially methylated) forms by biological systems. Not only are these methylated mercury compounds toxic, but highly bioaccumulative as well. [Mercury: A Factsheet For Healthcare Professionals. http://www.ingham.org/HD/LEPC/pamphlets/hazwaste/mercuryfacts.html]

Perhaps Dr. Haley says it simply and best:

If you have something that's been put in your mouth that you can't dispose of in a waste basket without breaking environmental protection laws, there's no point in keeping it around, there's no point in taking that type of risk - there's no point in exposing people to any level of mercury toxicity if you don't have to......[Dr. Boyd Haley, Professor of Medicinal Biochemistry, University of Kentucky, speaking on BBC Panorama]

Mercury Exposure Leads To A Damaged Immune System

Scientists routinely conduct studies in an effort to pinpoint that "one culprit" they can observe. The problem is that they rarely find the underlying, first and main culprit, like mercury, because it does its dirty work and then "hides". So science routinely finds all or many of the things going on and becomes confused. Indeed, until you understand the underlying role of mercury, you will never understand its widespread damage to DNA, mitochondria, kidneys, neurons, the immune system as a whole, etc. If you leave out the true culprit, you will never even begin to comprehend how any scientific discovery would factor in with regard to all the things going on in psoriasis.

For example, studies have shown that people with psoriasis test high for candida and other parasites (like strep). Scientists don't know why, but it's because the mercury-damaged immune system of a psoriatic isn't able to keep *any* virus, bacteria or fungus completely under control. So while scientists continue their studies, puzzled by the varied results, keep in mind that *mercury* caused the psoriasis – and everything else are all the "things going on". The goal, then, would be to eliminate any further mercury exposure and strengthen the immune system with natural, safe means.

If you think we're now safe from mercury because it's 2008, think again. Even though The Center for Disease Control states that there is **no acceptable amount of mercury that can enter your body,** you absorb and inhale mercury off of your "silver" fillings every day. In addition, if you go to the doctor, even in 2008, and get a flu shot or other immunization from a "multi-use" vial, there is still a liklihood it contains thimerosal (mercury used as the preservative). So how many "silver" fillings do you have?

"If they have more than four amalgam fillings in their mouth, the average person's saliva is so high in mercury they cannot legally spit in the toilet." [David Kennedy, DDS. Past President. International Academy of Oral Medicine and Toxicology. Davidkennedy-dds@ cox.net.]

Indeed, "silver fillings" don't contain much silver at all, but again, are over 50% mercury. Not only that, but there are toxic issues also with the copper, palladium and nickel also found in dental metals both combined with the mercury to make an "amalgam", and put under "gold" crowns.

Although it sometimes is called "silver **amalgam**," amalgam actually consists of a combination of silver, **mercury**, tin and copper, and small amounts of zinc, indium or palladium. [www.colgate.com]

The American Dental Association (obviously trying to avoid the massive lawsuits that would result from admission of guilt) still claims that the mercury in the tooth fillings is "inert" and does not enter your body. However there have been many tests done that have proven that fillings put mercury into the body. The International Academy of Oral Medicine and Toxicology created a video entitled *Smoking*

Teeth = Poison Gas. Mercury vapor is odorless, colorless and tasteless — but it casts a shadow in black light! This dramatic video of mercury vapor outgassing from an amalgam dental filling has outraged the world since it was first demonstrated in 1995. It is a *must see.* Simply type in Google: "Smoking Teeth = Poison Gas" and the video will come up on *You Tube.*

Caution: It is *not* recommended that you rush out to a regular "orthodox" dentist and request to have all of your amalgams removed. If they are removed incorrectly, you can actually overdose on mercury and make your situation worse rather than better (the video recommended above will explain this better than I can). You need to go to a genuine holistic dentist for proper removal. Ask someone you trust for a recommendation, or do some research by calling various "holistic" dentists and asking questions. Even if you choose not to have your existing tooth fillings removed, do not under any circumstances let your dentist add more mercury fillings to your teeth! The extra charge for a composite filling is usually very small and your continued health is more than worth that extra charge. **Composite fillings** are mercury free dental fillings that are also known as "white fillings".

Other Dangers Of Mercury

If you've ever questioned just how dangerous mercury is for your brain, there is a short film from the University of Calgary that will put your suspicions to rest. It is entitled *How Mercury Causes Brain Neuron Degeneration.* Again, Google that title and you will be taken to more than one site where you can watch this short video. Or type in: http://www.youtube.com/watch?v=IHqVDMr9ivo to go directly to the video on You Tube.

The video gets a little technical but you can ignore the technical parts and still understand perfectly why the mercury in tooth fillings or from any source is harmful and should be avoided. The film shows, in vivid detail, exactly what happens to your brain cells when they're exposed to mercury, making it easy to understand why mercury has been linked to a host of harmful reactions like candida, autism, heart disease, Parkinson's disease, multiple sclerosis, infertility and much more. (See Chapter 9 *Multiple Sclerosis* for a more thorough explanation of this video).

Mercury Has Been Around Since Before Christ

Mercury has been around for centuries. As previously mentioned, it has been found in Egyptian tombs proving that it was harnassed and used even before Christ. Evidence has been unearthed to find that India used mercury as a drug before Christ. Mercury came into use in America in the 18th century (1700s, when America was founded). The first known use was for syphilis. Mercury was also put into many other medicines such as antibacterial agents, for example, the aforementioned "mercurochrome". Today, every single American is exposed to mercury levels that exceed established health standards. But again, and this bears repeating ad nauseum: *There is no safe level of mercury.*

Scientists, even though they have conducted thousands of studies, have *not* been able to determine even one beneficial purpose served by the presence of this highly toxic metal in the human body. Absolutely no amount of exposure to mercury can be considered harmless. According to the CDC, mercury, along with lead and arsenic are the three most deadly substances on earth. Of course there are other highly toxic substances, like plutonium, radon or uranium, but they just don't exist to the degree of the aforementioned three. It is mercury that is by far the most prevalent in our world and bodies. Does it amaze you, as it does me, that *nobody would* think *to inject you with lead or arsenic!* So why in the heck have we been injected with mercury for all these years?

Unfortunately, mercury damage can go undetected for a person's entire lifetime! A person may suffer skin diseases, migraines, neurological disorders and depression, and doctors think they're all unrelated, and certainly never think of mercury as the cause! This is because mercury is "everywhere" and even brilliant doctors and scientists cannot believe that this ubiquitous substance can be causing so much havoc and suffering. What amazes me, is that when you walk into a doctor's office, the *last* thing on a doctor's mind is what could be causing your misery, your debilitation, your depression. The *first* thing on his mind is what test can he do to put a *name* to what you have, and then what drug can he prescribe to ameliorate your symptoms. It's a sad, sad state of affairs.

To complicate matters, the onset of a person's disease rarely comes instantly after being injected with mercury, or having an amalgam filling placed in their teeth. Bacteria in the mouth, stomach and intestines, or in the blood, through a process called *methylation*, converts mercury vapor and ionic mercury from ethylmercury into deadly *methylmercury*. According to the World Health Organization, 3-17 micrograms of mercury vapor is released into the body every day simply by chewing pressure on dental mercury fillings. The fact is, we do have all the puzzle pieces...we just can't seem to put them together fast enough or as clear as needed to save ourselves.

Considerable damage can occur, however, **if mercury is made airborne** into small, little droplets and breathed into the lungs. This can often occur by mistake when people try to vacuum up mercury that has spilled onto the ground. Breathing in elemental mercury will cause symptoms right away (acute) if enough mercury is breathed in. Symptoms will also occur over time (chronic) if little amounts are inhaled every day. Depending on how much mercury is inhaled, permanent lung damage and death may occur. You may also have some long-term brain damage from inhaled elemental mercury. [http://www2.healthtalk.com]

Where Else Is All The Mercury Coming From?

Mercury is used by many industries, such as in the manufacturing of batteries, thermometers, barometers and more. Manufacturers dump their wastes into our waterways and the fish swimming in those waters absorb the mercury and pass it along to you when you eat the fish. Mercury wastes can also get into our landfills, seeping down into the water table and then into our water supply. And now manufacturers and your precious government are pushing "long-life" light bulbs which contain mercury! If you break one of those bulbs and simply sweep it up, you're breathing in highly toxic mercury! When you throw that bulb into the trash, as many millions will, that mercury ends up in our landfills, spilling their mercury into the soil and down into the water table.

Hmmm. I know of several people who either died or are dying from lung cancer – and they never smoked. In fact, there seems to be a bit of an epidemic of lung cancer in people who have never smoked. In addition, mercury is used in many fungicides used in spraying crops. Prior to 1990 paints even contained mercury as an antimildew agent!

It wasn't until July of 1999 that the American Academy of Pediatrics and the US Public Health Service issued an alert to physicians as to the "possible" danger of thimerosal (contains ethylmercury which we've seen ends up in the brain) in their vaccines. But as late as 2006, thimerosal can still be found in vaccines. I shared before about how my granddaughter was born September, 2006, and there was thimerosal in the hepatitis B vaccine they tried to give her just minutes after she was born! *I'll be forever grateful I was there to stop this.* She is today, the most beautiful, healthy child, *free* of all of the many childhood ailments so prevalent today.

Mercury Destroys Everything In Its Path

Mercury easily vaporizes at room temperature and is readily absorbed through skin or inhalation. It passes easily through the lung's alveoli and into the bloodstream and thus into the red blood cells. Mercury causes central nervous system damage. In fact, mercury is associated with over 200 different symptoms, and copper, also found in amalgam, with over 100. The severe toxicity of methylmercury is attributed to its ability to penetrate your cell membranes as well as cross all your natural barriers, such as the placental and blood-brain barriers. After crossing these barriers, methylmercury is converted back into the highly destructive ionic form which destroys all cell components in its path. In fact, mercury vapor easily crosses the blood-brain barrior where it is trapped, causing serious damage to neurons and the central nervous system. It is this damage, depending upon where in the brain the damage occurs, how much mercury did the damage, and how widespread the damage is, that dictates the type of neurological disease that ensues, and the severity. So it's not just skin diseases like psoriasis, but also Alzheimer's, Parkinson's, multiple sclerosis, autism, depression and more that are caused by mercury.

If mercury could be completely and forever eliminated, we would likely find in just a few short years, many diseases virtually *disappear*. Mercury toxicity, by virtue of its cellular and neurotoxicity has been implicated as well, in anorexia, diabetes, fatigue, insomnia, arthritis, irritability, memory loss, any chronic infection, migraines, and so much more. Even before birth, since mercury easily crosses the placental barrier, its toxicity could easily cause cerebral palsy, retardation or any of a number of "birth defects". With what I now know *and have personally experienced* about mercury, I now know that a "birth defect" is really a *mutation* to genes by toxic materials within the parent (or grandparent or great-grandparent, etc.). The toxic substance likely doing most of the mutating since B.C., is mercury.

After The Damage Comes The Parasites

Psoriasis can be provoked or exacerbated by a variety of different environmental factors, particularly infections and drugs. Strong evidence exists for the induction of guttate psoriasis by a preceding tonsillar **Streptococcus** pyogenes infection, whereas disease exacerbation has been linked with skin and/or gut colonization by Staphylococcus aureus, Malassezia, and **Candida albicans**. [*Clin Dermatol* 2007 Nov-Dec;25(6):606-15.]

The fungus *Candida albicans* has long been linked to psoriasis. It didn't "cause" psoriasis, mercury did. But *Candida* is involved in the perpetuation of the antigens (foreign particles) that get into the bloodstream and end up as psoriasis (inflammation, exudation). *Candida* both flourishes in and damages the entire GI tract. Once *Candida* establishes a strong foothold, it grows and imbeds itself into the lining of the GI tract. It's byproducts spew into the bloodstream as does more *Candida*, causing a "systemic" (bodywide) infection. This can be chronic — even persisting a person's entire lifetime (especially since doctors aren't looking for it). Some symptoms of the presence of *Candida* (called "candidiasis") are vaginal yeast, thrush, fingernails lifted, yellowed toe and fingernails, gas, and bloating but also so much more — including any number of inflammatory and exudative skin diseases.

Ironically, *Candida* has been shown to absorb mercury. The body can increase the growth of yeast in the gut to absorb mercury as a sort of natural "sponge". Then, the trapped mercury catalyzes oxidative damage, damaging the gut even further, preventing nutrients from entering cells and wastes from leaving by blocking enzymes necessary for the body's natural detoxification. Mercury damages the cell's DNA (genetic material) as well as the cell's membrane causing altered cell membrane permeability. This damage makes normal cell functioning impossible. The damage is also to cells that make up the immune system, i.e., that system that protects the body from foreign invaders. The body is now less able to eliminate wastes properly. The damage can also lead to "autoimmune" problems wherein the immune system becomes "confused" and turns around and attacks the body itself. These are *all the things going on* in psoriasis. But, again, the *cause* was mercury.

Psoriasis Is *Caused* By Mercury

Dr. Paul I. Dantzig, M.D., Department of Dermatology at Columbia University, School of Medicine reports on **a 31-year old white female who suddenly erupted with psoriais.** All blood tests were normal, except:

> …blood mercury was 22 micrograms/Liter. Patient was begun on fluocinonide ointment, a strict no seafood diet and succimer 300 mg TID which resulted in a cessation of new lesions and a marked decrease in inflammation of older lesions and a lowering a blood mercury. [email Dr. Dantzig at pid@drmercury.com - Paul Dantzig MD is a Board Certified Dermatologist and received his medical degree from George Washington University, Washington D.C. in 1971]

PSORIASIS

This patient erupted suddenly. Others with psoriasis may never be tested for mercury, so the relationship might not be discovered. Then there will be patients who are tested for mercury, but tested incorrectly (mercury doesn't hang around in the blood awaiting testing, as previously explained) and so a false assumption that mercury plays no role would be made.

Dr. Dantzig goes on to say that finding that mercury causes guttae psoriasis is important because it provides physicians with not only the ability to then properly treat patients, but also with the basis to then help other people *prevent* psoriasis. In addition, knowing what causes psoriasis provides the basis upon which we can continue research to discern *how* mercury ends up causing the symptoms of inflammation and exudation we call psoriasis. Why I reiterate this, is because I find it surprisingly honest and wise coming from a person trained to administer drugs. There are approximately 200 physicians in the U.S. per 100,000 population. How many of them are looking for the underlying *cause* of a disease so they can properly treat it, help people prevent it, and even aim their future research in all the right directions? I've known dozens of doctors, and only met maybe one who even came close to this.

The Most Important Things You Can Do

It's no coincidence that children are the ones who usually come down with psoriasis first. This is because psoriasis will occur after that mouthful of amalgams or batch of immunizations children are more likely to receive than adults. The gut and immune system are badly damaged by mercury leaving a body to fight far more "antigens" than it was ever designed to fight. The earlier you begin to incorporate healing measures, the better. No child should have to grow up feeling like a leper.

First – No more mercury from any source of course! No amalgams and no immunizations containing mercury (or aluminum, formaldehyde, etc.). It's your call whether or not you want to use immunizations that say they do not contain thimerosal, but please do your homework as to the true need for them as well as to what other toxins might be in that vial. You can get a lot of excellent information at www.mercola.com. Put in a search for articles on immunizations, mercury, and thimerosal. Be sure to listen to his 2008 call to the vaccine company wherein it was admitted that vaccines still contain mercury, even if they say they don't! Search for: "Do Flu Shots Work? Ask a Vaccine Manufacturer".

Also, no fish consumption unless you're truly out in the wilderness somewhere and caught your own from fresh, clean waters! Most oceans, seas and lakes are polluted, and factories are spewing more pollutants into the waters daily. Its just not worth the risk. Consume mostly organic plant foods, but include some organic eggs and poultry for satisfying any desire for animal protein. Get your essential fatty acids the same way many animals do, by consuming copious quantities of greens.

Second – The best way to deal topically with psoriasis is this: Thoroughly cover the scales with an emollient like the aforementioned Dermarest. There is no magic to the cream. The idea is that it softens the scales. Then when you shower or bathe, the scales can be rubbed off right down to the skin, and you'll feel so much more human.

Third – There has been a lot of publicity about the benefit of sunshine for the Vitamin D. For psoriatics sunshine is doubly essential. What actually causes the healing of psoriasis exposed to sunshine is **sweating** and internal factors (likely from the vitamin D). This is why a suntan salon won't do the trick. You may darken/tan the skin or even burn it and it will appear that the psoriasis has lessened, but *nothing* works like natural sunlight and sweat.

Fourth – You must **avoid any form of "fiberless sugars" and carrageenan.** These contribute to the overgrowth of *Candida* already present and contributing hugely to the problem of psoriasis. This means no corn syrup, honey, white sugar, "fructose" etc. as found in cans, jars and products. You can, however, have a normal amount of fresh, whole fruits in your daily diet. In fact, the natural sugars are *essential* to feed the "good guys" you want to flourish in your GI tract so they can become your internal army – digesting food as well as fighting off bad bacteria and fungus.

Fifth Never use cortisone creams or oral cortisone medications. If you try them you'll find that your psoriasis clears right up — but then returns worse than before. Cortisone applied topically is absorbed systemically and will cause a worsening of viral and fungal infections. Oral cortisone eats away at the stomach and intestinal lining, causing ulcerations.

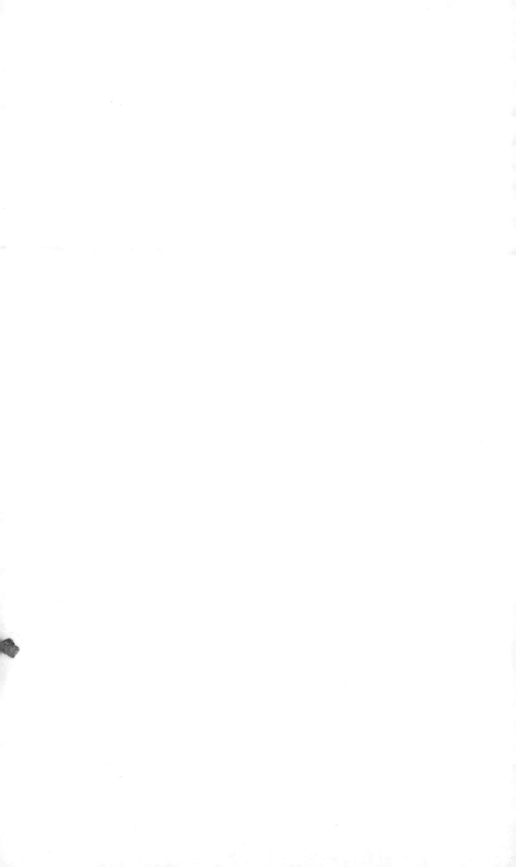

Chapter 8
MIGRAINES

After reading, you should understand that if you had never been damaged by **mercury**, you would not have migraines; how the **glutamatergic system** has been damaged which means your body cannot break down or properly use glutamate (thus **dietary free glutamates/excitotoxins** must be banned forever); how excess glutamate leads to excess **nitric oxide** which is the molecule that sparks the **neurological firestorm** that is a migraine; how there are "many things going on" that confound even doctors and scientists and keep you from obtaining the truth to motivate you to do what you need to do (as well as prevent migraines in future generations); and how **dangerous drugs** are *not* the answer.

Mercury Is The Underlying *Cause* Of Migraines

The *cause* of migraines, again, the pollutant (see Chapter 5 *All The Things Going On*) initially is **mercury**. Mercury causes heavy metal damage to the brain, immune system, and glutamatergic system. This explains why men, women and children all get migraines. It explains why even people since the beginning of time are known to have had migraines. Indeed, man has been harnassing and using heavy metals since ancient days. In fact, mercury was known to ancient Chinese and Hindus before 2000 B.C. and was found in tubes in Egyptian tombs dated as early as 1500 B.C.

We know today that mercury is a virulent poison and is readily absorbed through the respiratory tract, gastrointestinal tract, or through unbroken skin. In spite of what ignorant (meaning unaware of the truth) people say, mercury acts as a cumulative poison since there are few pathways available in the body for its complete excretion. It baffles me how on earth mercury, after the discoveries centuries ago, ever got approved to be put on skin sores, injected directly into the body (thimerosal in flu and other vaccines) or into teeth ("amalgam" fillings, and thereby put into the body permanently). Again, we've known about mercury's horrific toxicity for hundreds of years! I have to ask...are we really *that* stupid?

Consider these people, who knew in the 16th to the 18th century that mercury causes horrific damage to the human body. Note that the name Huguenot was applied to a member of the Protestant Reformed Church of France.

> "The Huguenots (c. 16ᵗʰ-18ᵗʰ century) did the English hatters no favor by sharing their secret with them. The pelts were usually dipped into the hot mercuric nitrate in poorly ventilated rooms and so common were the symptoms of mercurialism that terms such as "the hatters' shakes" and "mad as a hatter" passed into everyday speech. The pyschotic symptoms of mercury poisoning had been described during the eighteenth century when mercurial ointments were used in the treatment of syphilis." [See: http://www.pubmedcentral.nih.gov/pagerender.fcgi?artid=1550196&pageindex=1]

Today, mercury is number *three* on the Center for Disease Control's list of the most poisonous substances on earth (following arsenic and lead). With regard to migraines, **studies show that because of mercury damage, the brain's ability to properly utilize glutamate leads to a cascade of events the most harmful of which is the excess**

production of nitric oxide which ultimately leads to the neurological firestorm that is a migraine.

After reading literally thousands of studies, it is clear to me that if there are many factors involved in coming up with a single answer, brilliant men and women just don't seem to have the sense or notion to put all those factors together. I find that most scientists remain focused on their one little piece of the puzzle. In their defense, it is true that mercury doesn't instantly cause a migraine necessarily, but is the damaging culprit which eventually causes a person to become a "migraineur". So even I can see where coming up with the "cause" of migraines might be complex. But here we are, centuries after it was clearly known how horribly neurotoxic mercury is, with dentists still packing it into people's teeth, and doctor's still injecting it into people's arms! I've come to the conclusion that often our most important discoveries come from a single, determined individual, not men and women in labs. Consider the following.

If I were to walk into my kitchen every Tuesday night and a pot falls out of an upper cupboard and onto my head, I might think this is an accident – the first time. But if *every* Tuesday night a pot falls out of an upper cupboard onto my head, I might realize that this is something that happens on Tuesday nights, and I need to either fix the cupboard, take that pot out of the cupboard, or avoid walking under it that night, at that time. I could then share with everyone about Tuesday, about the cupboard, and about the pot. Or, if I *simply removed the pot* I would solve the problem. History shows us that scientists will spend dozens of years studying the aerodynamics of the pot falling, the type of pot, why on a Tuesday and not Wednesday, other cupboards to see if they have pots in them, not just the shaking that caused the cupboard to release that pot, but the magnitude of the shaking, etc. Unfortunately, with that method these brilliant minds *rarely* conclude to simply remove the pot and spare everyone the damage and misery of being hit on the head every Tuesday night. And so it is with mercury.

What follows is an overview of what *really* causes a migraine. You can come back to it all later if you like after you get a better idea of all the particulars. I believe all the science needs to be included - you've been kept in the dark too long! In a nutshell, mercury damages systems that involve the production, use and recycling of *glutamate*, the most prevalent neurotransmitter, responsible for the "synapsing" (connecting) of neurons. When glutamates are out of control, neurons fire wildly, unpredictably, and even die. Migraines are caused by a "neurological firestorm" i.e., *neurons behaving badly, wildly, excessively.* . . .

MERCURY DAMAGES THE GLUTAMATERGIC SYSTEM

The present study clearly demonstrates that **(mercury) inhibited glutamate uptake** in human platelets. The present limited results could suggest that glutamatergic system may be used as a potential biomarker for neurotoxic action of heavy metals in humans. [*Neurochem Res* 2007 Jun;32(6):953-8.] **Alterations of the neurotransmitter release systems** (e.g., glutamatergic system) in the central nervous system have been reported in a variety of neuropathological processes associated with **heavy metal toxicity**. Neurotoxic effects of mercurials were investigated. [*Toxicology* Volume 214, Issues 1-2, 15 October 2005, Pages 57-66]

A DAMAGED GLUTAMATERGIC SYSTEM CAN'T PROCESS GLUTAMATE, SO EXCESS GLUTAMATE CAUSES OVERACTIVATION OF COMPOUNDS THAT LEAD TO EXCESS NITRIC OXIDE [in this study referred to as "oxygen free radicals"]

Because of **a damaged glutamatergic system** the person is ultra sensitive to toxic dietary free glutamates, or precursors to glutamate release, or the body's own release of the excitatory neurotransmitter glutamate. **The excess glutamates causes a neurological firestorm:** ischemia, increases in intracellular calcium levels, over-activation of different protein kinases and triggers enzyme reactions which finally result in excessive production of oxygen free radicals, damage of cell membranes, inflammation and **PAIN** (such as a migraine) and ultimately neuronal death. [Birgit Hutter-Paier et al *Journal of Neural Transmission* Volume 113, Number 1 , January, 2006 P.103-110]

EXCESSIVE GLUTAMATE → NITRIC OXIDE (Oxygen Free Radicals) LEAD TO THE DEATH OF NEURONS, AND IS TOXIC TO WHITE MATTER CAUSING WHITE MATTER LESIONS SEEN IN BOTH MIGRAINES AND MS

Glutamate kills neurons by excitotoxicity, which is caused by sustained activation of glutamate receptors. In recent years, it has been shown that **glutamate can also be toxic to white matter** oligodendrocytes and to myelin by this mechanism. [C. Matute et al White matter injury by glutamate March 6, 2007]

NITRIC OXIDE AND SUPEROXIDE COMBINE TO FORM A MORE TOXIC PRODUCT

Nitric oxide and superoxide are free radicals that appear to contribute to the pathogenesis of a number of brain disorders. Enhanced levels of **superoxide can combine with nitric oxide** to form a more toxic product. [*Pharmacology and Experimental Therapeutics* Vol. 282, Issue 3, 1600-1607, 1997]

ESTROGEN PEAKING CAUSES RELEASE OF LEUTENIZING HORMONE WHICH STIMULATES RELEASE OF GLUTAMATE → Nitric Oxide

When estrogen reaches its peak in the female cycle it causes an abrupt release of leutenizing hormone which is the hormone that triggers ovulation. There is a simultaneous **increase during this time of the excitatory amino acid neurotransmitters aspartate and glutamate** in the preoptic/anterior hypothalamic area of the brain. [*Neuroendocrinology* 1992 Aug;56(2):133-40.]

TOXIC LEVELS OF GLUTAMATE CAUSE NITRIC OXIDE TO BE RELEASED IN AN ATTEMPT TO MEDIATE THE EXCESS GLUTAMATE

When toxic levels of glutamate are released, nitric oxide is released in response. Nitric oxide tries to mediate the neurotoxicity of glutamate [V L Dawson et al Neuropharmacology Laboratory, National Institute on Drug Abuse Addiction Research Center, Baltimore, MD 21224.]

NITRIC OXIDE IS A POTENT VASODILATOR AND SPARKS THE CASCADE OF EVENTS THAT ENDS IN THE NEUROLOGICAL FIRESTORM, VASODILATATION AND INFLAMMATION THAT IS A MIGRAINE

Nitric oxide is a potent vasodilator and triggers the neurological firestorm that is a migraine. [Ideggyogy Sz. 2006 Nov 20;59 (11-12):389-95]

The previously reported observation that submicromolar concentrations of HgCl2 **mercury inhibits glutamate uptake** reversibly in astrocytes, without effect on 2-deoxyglucose uptake, suggested that elemental mercury vapor, which is oxidized to mercuric mercury in the brain, might cause **neurodegenerative change** through the **mediation of glutamate excitotoxicity**. The first published report of human adverse reactions to "processed free glutamic acid" appeared in *The New England Journal of Medicine* in 1968. [N. Brookes et al. Inhibition of Amino Acid Transport and Protein Synthesis by HgCl2 and Methylmercury in Astrocytes: Selectivity and Reversibility. *Journal of Neurochemistry* 53 (4), 1228–1237. 1989.]

A Migraine Is A Neurological Firestorm

It has been proposed that **mercury** exposure **inhibits astroglial ability to take up glutamate**, leading to glutamate receptor hypersensitivity, decreased cortical glutamate, and secondary decreases in other neurotransmitters. Decreased activity in the locus coeruleus will lead to symptoms reported by patients with low-dose exposures, e.g., fatigue and decreased alertness (Rönnbäck & Hansson, 1992). At higher concentrations, extracellular glutamate may become toxic to neurons. [Neuropsychological Toxicology By David E. Hartman 1995]

Mercury damages the brain's ability to handle glutamates by damaging the ability of glutamates to be broken down and reprocessed, keeping glutamate from excessive buildup. This is part of the glutamatergic system, called the glutamate transport system.

Calcitonin gene related peptide CGRP, **nitric oxide** NO and cytokines are all molecules shown to be involved both in animal and human studies. The **glutamatergic system** is also described as a possible mechanism leading to **neuronal hyperexcitability**. [Longoni M et al. Inflammation and excitotoxicity: role in **migraine** pathogenesis. *Neurol Sci.* 2006 May;27 Suppl 2:S107-10.]

Damaging The Glutamate Transport System Is Only Done By Mercury

Mercury causes damage to the neuron's ability to gather up and reprocess glutamate via the "glutamatergic transport system", and researchers have found that this is something **unique to mercury**. When researchers attempted to elicit the same response from other metals, like copper or zinc, they found inhibition of glutamate uptake to be specific only to mercury. [P. Kim et al Selective Inhibition of Glutamate uptake by mercury in cultured mouse astrocytes, Yonsel Medical Journal, Vol. 36 No. 3, 1995.]

As mentioned above, the glutamate transporters' job is to "recycle" the glutamate, that is, break it down and reuse it. Instead, glutamate builds up (both because of the damaged glutamatergic system, and the sheer excess of glutamates in the normal diet) and causes a series of events leading to a migraine as well as damage, even death to neurons. This is why a damaged glutamatergic system isn't merely a concern of migraineurs. Indeed, *all neurological diseases involve neuron damage*, from excess glutamate and the events following its excessive release.

I'll pause here and leave you with a thought. If you find it difficult to believe that so many diseases can stem from one nasty perpetrator, let's revisit the *Fall of the Roman Empire.* In approximately A.D. 476 the Roman Empire has been said to have "fallen" or ceased to exist as a viable society. Like so many historical events, controversy over the reasons for the fall have existed for centuries. Controversy or not, in the end, there were virtually few people left. Here are some of the proposed reasons:

> There are adherents to single factors, but more people think Rome fell because of a combination of such factors as Christianity, decadence, **lead**, monetary trouble, and military problems. Even the rise of Islam is proposed as the reason for Rome's fall...[http://ancienthistory.about.com/cs/romefallarticles/a/fallofrome.htm]

While religious views, decadence, monetary trouble and military problems are all problems humans have faced throughout history – they are the same problems we face today. They do great damage, but rarely wipe out an entire society. The most toxic and far-reaching of the possible problems is "lead" as in heavy metal, one of the three most toxic substances man foolishly harnesses and chooses to use in his daily life. Recall that they decided to make their entire drinking water pipe system out of lead. *Everyone would have ultimately been poisoned.* So you can speculate all you want. With what's going on with mercury today, I *know* what caused the fall of Rome.

So, the answer is yes, we *can* point to mercury as the single underlying cause of an entire group of diseases. Neurological diseases all have mercury as the underlying perpetrator, as likely do autoimmune diseases, diabetes, and cancer. Likewise, *all* of these diseases go on to involve a defect in the glutamatergic transport system and thus glutamate buildup which then causes neurons to fire uncontrollably and die, among other things.

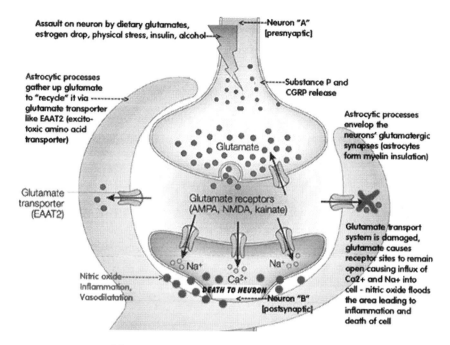

Neurons Synapsing, note the glutamate release

As depicted in the diagram above, some of the assaults to neurons that lead to excess glutamate release are the peaking and then drop of estrogen, excessive visual or other stimuli (in fact studies have found excess glutamate in the brain of babies in "shaken baby syndrome"). Consumption of alcohol leads to excess glutamate release, as does, of course the consumption of free glutamates found in all our processed and packaged foods. Ultimately, then, excess glutamates cause *excess nitric oxide* **leading** to the neurological firestorm that is a migraine.

So, the first and most important step for a migraineur is to accept that *any* amount of free glutamates you consume in your foods is "in excess", as you aren't meant to consume *any*. Glutamate in nature is "bound", not free. I've seen lists where they show whole, natural foods having "glutamates". For example you'll find peas, tomatoes, and milk on that list. This is very deceiving. The "bound" glutamate in those foods is harmless. Only the "free glutamates" (meaning, not bound to anything) are harmful to the body. Free glutamates are created by processing proteins using procedures such as fermentation, hydrolyzation, enzymes, texturization, and isolation.

Persistent Over-Activation Of Synaptic Glutamate Receptors

Because of mercury's damage to the neural system of glutamate transport, eventually the body develops a state of "chronic overexcitation". Where it used to take a high glutamate meal three days to cause symptoms, now there is hypersensitivity to even the smallest amount. It is not uncommon to hear of people who have migraines one, two, even three times per week.

The present study indicates that **defective** spinal **glutamate uptake caused by inhibition of glutamate transporters** leads to excessive glutamate accumulation in the spinal cord. The latter results in **persistent over-activation** of synaptic glutamate receptors, producing spontaneous nociceptive (responds to painful or noxious stimuli) behaviors and sensory **hypersensitivity**. [Liaw Wen-Jinn et al *Pain* 2005, vol. 115, no 1-2, pp. 60-70]

Why isn't all this front page news?

Likely because the great minds that discover these individual findings in laboratories or clincial studies don't quite know what to do with the information. This is especially true when they have many bits and pieces of information, which haven't been put together into one clear picture. In addition, and as previously mentioned, to say "mercury did the damage" opens up a floodgate of lawsuit potential from all those who are suffering (about 2 out of every 3 people – from one neurological disease or another).

Unfortunately scientific studies are also funded by entities that are looking for multi-million dollar income from their discoveries. So to simply say, "don't consume any dietary glutamates" as an initial course of action doesn't lead to any drug to stop "all the things going on".

There goes millions if not billions of income to doctors, hospitals, laboratories, scientists, and pharmaceutical companies. While not all scientific investigation has a new drug and multi-millions in profits as their goal, all too many *do*. I believe this next story sums up what can happen when money is the motive for the discoveries.

In the news August 2008, a scientist, Bruce Ivins, commited suicide. He had been discovered to be the person who, in 2001, had mailed anthrax to the Senate building. Why? Well, this scientist had been working on an anthrax vaccine. But then the scare had died down. In order to ensure that his work (and income) continued, he mailed anthrax out (resulting in the death of five people and terror to us all) so that the nation would *insist* upon coming up with a good vaccine. So you think scientists would never keep important discoveries from you that could alleviate your suffering? This illustration is extreme, of course. However, in many smaller ways, yes, you might be kept in the dark, if by giving you the truth, those who stand to make so much money would have their research (and income) stopped.

How Mercury Damages the Glutamatergic System

We now know that mercury damages the brain's glutamatergic system *irreversibly* because we know it damages DNA and the mitochondria of cells.

> We studied the prevalence, segregation, and phenotype of the **mitochondrial DNA 3243A>G mutation** in children in a defined population in Northern Ostrobothnia, Finland. The first clinical manifestations appearing in childhood were sensorineural hearing impairment, short stature or delayed maturation, **migraine**, learning difficulties, and exercise intolerance. [Löppönen T et al. Prevalence, segregation, and phenotype of the mitochondrial DNA 3243A>G mutation in children. *Ann Neurol.*2007 Sep 6;62(3):278-287]

DNA contains the genetic instructions used in the development and functioning of all known living organisms. DNA molecules are like your cell's blueprint (instructions) for building different structures as well as orchestrating functions. Armed with just that information alone, you can see what can happen if your DNA is damaged! Things go haywire. Below is a study your doctor won't share with you prior to giving you a flu shot containing mercury.

Mercury is a xenobiotic metal that is well known to **adversely affect the immune system...** we found that **mercury damaged DNA** [E. Y. Ben-Ozer et al. Mercuric chloride damages cellular DNA by a non-apoptotic mechanism. Institute of Chemical Toxicology, Wayne State University, Detroit, MI 48202, USA. June 2000.]

Note that the glutamatergic system is made up of cells that must function properly and *not* have damaged DNA or mitochondria. The mitochondria are rod-shaped organelles within all your cells, except your red blood cells, and are responsible for energy production. Mitochondria also contain a small amount of DNA. Again, impaired mitochondria is involved in migraines and mercury does the impairing. The study at the bottom of this page talks of "mutations", which we now know are caused by mercury.

...impaired mitochondrial energy metabolism in migraine. [*P. Montagna* Mitochondrial Abnormalities in Migraine. Preliminary Findings. Congress of the Italian Neurological Society, Bologna, 1987]

Refer again to the first textbox on this page. As previously mentioned, only by stringing together all the findings of various studies can we put together all the puzzle pieces to get a clear picture.

Mutations associated with familial hemiplegic migraine render the brain more susceptible to prolonged cortical spreading depression caused by either **excessive synaptic glutamate** release or **decreased removal of glutamate.** In all cases the final consequence leads to mechanisms that support the **hyperexcitability of the migraineur brain.** [New insights into migraine pathophysiology. Lippincott Williams & Wilkins, Inc. Volume 19(3), June 2006, p 294–298]

Excess glutamate activity is something migraneurs share:

Recent advances have shed insight on the pathophysiologic mechanisms of...migraines... **increased glutamate transmission**... increased levels of glutamate in the cerebrospinal fluid of affected patients... [Sarchielli P et al. Sensitization, glutamate, and the link between migraine and fibromyalgia. *Curr Pain Headache Rep.* 2007 Oct;11(5):343-51.]

When you have increased glutamate transmission, you have an increase release of nitric oxide production (the direct precursor to a migraine).

In addition to mediating several physiological functions, **nitric oxide (NO)** has been implicated in the cytotoxicities observed **following activation of macrophages or excess stimulation of neurons by glutamate.** [*Journal of Neuroscience,* Vol 13, 2651-2661, 1993]

What Exactly Is The Glutamatergic System?

The glutamatergic neurotransmitter system is how neurons synapse in your brain and central nervous sytem. Neurons carry information from the brain and central nervous system to the rest of your body, like your muscles and internal organs. When neurons synapse properly (completely, not too excitedly, nor too lazily, etc), you have proper memory and processing of information and mood. Also when your neurons synapse properly, you find everything behaving within the brain and central nervous sytstem, which means you *don't* have excessive inflammation, vasodilatation or vasoconstriction. Glutamate is the most common "excitatory" neurotransmitter in the central nervous system.

Not all neurotransmitters are equally important. By far the most prevalent transmitter is glutamate, which is used at well over 90% of the synapses in the human brain. [From Wikipedia]

A tiny little bit of glutamate is required for the firing of neurons, and *your body makes all it needs.* Consuming *any* in the diet is excessive.

Healthy people can handle the excess for a while, but if continued *all* people will ultimately have some degree of brain damage – especially given we're all exposed to mercury! For migraineurs the glutamatergic sytem has been damaged *badly* so that the slightest provocation causes a devastating cascade of events that lead to a neurological firestorm ultimately causing the inflammation and horrific pain of a migraine. For people who don't suffer the pain of migraine, the neurological firestorm (happening to a different degree or in different areas of the brain and body) cause other horrific outcomes:

Just a few examples:

1) *Rev Neurol* 2006 Apr 1-15;42(7):427-32. Glutamate and Alzheimer's disease. CONCLUSION: **Glutamatergic dysfunction** plays an important role in the pathogenesis of this illness.

2) *Mol Neurobiology* 1996 Feb;12(1):73-94. Glutamate and Parkinson's disease. The involvement of the **glutamatergic system** in the pathogenesis and symptomatology of PD provides potential new targets for therapeutic intervention in this neurodegenerative disorder.

3) *Nature Medicine* 6, 67-70 (2000) Glutamate excitotoxicity in a model of multiple sclerosis Glutamate **excitotoxicity** mediated by the AMPA/kainate type of glutamate receptors damages not only neurons but also the myelin-producing cell of the central nervous system, the oligodendrocyte.

4) *Free Radic Biol Med.* 2007 Jan 1;42(1):143-51. Amyotrophic lateral sclerosis (**ALS**) is an adult-onset neurodegenerative disorder in which **excitotoxicity** has been implicated as a cause for cell death.

5) *Macular Degeneration* by P Penfold and J Provis 2005. "The collective **changes** that we describe **in the glutamate transport system** suggest that there are significant imbalances in the homeostasis of glutamate in the AMD (age-related macular degeneration) retina. We suggest that the novel

expression of GLT-I in the retinal ganglion cells (which has never before been described) may be induced in response to **elevated extracellular glutamate levels** concomitant with the down-regulation of GLAST. This perturbation of glutamate homeostasis may also explain why retinal ganglion cells have been observed to die in AMD.

6) Epilepsy *Am J Hum Genet.* 2005 February; 76(2): 334–339. **patient cells failed to normally oxidize glutamate. These results provide evidence that patient cells show a clear defect in mitochondrial glutamate metabolism.**

7) "Researchers have observed abnormally high levels of **glutamate** in people and animals with glaucoma. Glutamate is an amino acid that excites nerve cells. In the eye this occurs during vision. Some experts theorize that in glaucoma, either reduced blood flow or increased pressure on nerve cells triggers the release of excess glutamate. In large amounts, glutamate causes the nerve cells to fire intensively, which eventually destroys them." [http://www.umm.edu/patiented/articles/what_causes_glaucoma_optic_nerve_damage_000025_2.htm]

I believe we will find the presence of a damaged glutamatergic system in every neurological disease known to man, and it shouldn't surprise anyone. Mercury is highly toxic, *everyone* is exposed because dentists pack it into teeth and doctors inject it into bodies daily. But the exposure doesn't end there. The possible sources are endless and range from mercury put into cosmetics to breathing it because of living near crematoriums or other industries spewing it into the environment, to fish polluted from mercury in our oceans, lakes and streams. The more exposure, the more damage done to the body and neurological system. Why one person gets Parkinson's and another gets multiple sclerosis has to do with where in the body the mercury damage has occurred, as well as any inherent weaknesses or previous damage.

Psychologists will tell you that attention-deficit hyperactivity disorder, obsessive-compulsive disorder, clinical depression and other mood disorders are also as a result of damage to the **glutamatergic system**. But I haven't found any doctors yet that have put the puzzle pieces together and announced that mercury is the initial culprit. It is becoming clearer that *not* announcing mercury as the initial culprit has a lot to do with doctors' fear to admit that they themselves *caused* the problem by their mercury-containing medicines and dental materials.

Excess Glutamate Causes White Matter Lesions

Animal feeding studies done by independent researchers have demonstrated that **"processed free glutamic acid" causes brain lesions** in the area of the **hypothalamus**. [Kwok, R.H.M. Chinese restaurant syndrome. *New England Journal of Medicine,* 17:796, 1968]

Excess glutamate causes white matter lesions on the brain. These are "diseased" areas in the brain. It is possible that it is from these very lesions migraines *eminate* as they are weakened areas where the series of events leading to a neurological firestorm could occur. While there are many powerful things a migraineur can do to stop the neurological firestorm, likely the only complete healing will happen when you can go to your doctor and get **neural stem cells** injected right into the damaged part of your brain (more on that later).

White matter is one of the three main solid components of the central nervous system. The other two are gray matter and substantia nigra. White matter is composed of myelinated nerve cell processes which connect various gray matter areas of the brain to each other and carry nerve impulses between neurons.

You might want to have an MRI to see if you have "white matter lesions". However, because damage by mercury and then by glutamates is so prevalent, doctors reading your MRI may say that your white matter lesions are "normal" and possibly due to your age. Again, that's because most people have some degree of white matter lesions. Of course they do! Everyone is exposed to mercury, and everyone consume free glutamates. Many people are also getting neurological disorders whether frequent headaches, migraines, Parkinson's or the beginnings of Alzheimer's. White matter lesions are <u>not</u> "normal", but pathological.

Glutamate kills neurons by excitotoxicity, which is caused by sustained activation of glutamate receptors. In recent years, it has been shown that glutamate can also be **toxic to white matter oligodendrocytes and to myelin by this mechanism**. Excitotoxic cell death can occur in virtually all neurons which express ionotropic glutamate receptors (GluRs) and it has been implicated in acute injury to the central nervous system (CNS) and in chronic neurodegenerative disorders [Choi, 1988; Lipton & Rosenberg, 1994; Lee et al. 1999].

Migraineurs can have damage to areas of the brain other than the hypothalamus. My own white matter lesions were found in the right frontal and left femoral lobes. Every time I discover something about my own migraines, somewhere, a scientific discovery is made connecting the dots for me. I had the MRI in August of 2006. Here in 2008 I read:

Neuroimaging studies have identified **frontal lobe brain** abnormalities in migraineurs. [*Neuroscience Letters* Volume 440, Issue 2, August 1, 2008, Pages 92-96]

Excessive glutamate activity in the hypothalamus is being observed, and does tie in to the mechanism of a migraine – a *neurological firestorm*.

A French team observed activation in the **hypothalamus** region of the brain as sufferers had a migraine attack. [BBC News December 25, 2007 Arran Frood]

If you do decide to have an MRI be forwarned that it's expensive and a bit frightening, but you only need to do the brain. I had a full body MRI in one day and would never do it again. It was the latest

Tesla machine and I was a busy person wanting to get it over with in a day. They did the brain, cervical spine, lumbar and thoracic area.... three different MRIs, each taking about 10-15 minutes. By the time they got to the lower back I felt like I was being cooked, literally. It was frighteningly hot, and I had to lie still for a long time. How much damage did that do to my body? I'll never know. However, my results were that I have two areas of "white matter lesions", and one of the areas is at the exact "epicenter" of the migraines I've suffered for over 20 years.

> ....a high prevalence of silent lesions was found in the posterior circulation resembling small infarcts. [New insights into migraine pathophysiology. Lippincott Williams & Wilkins, Inc. Volume 19(3), June 2006, p 294–298]

It bears repeating: *Lesions on brain white matter are caused by "free glutamates"* which are being put into our processed and packaged foods by the metric tons every single year. The white matter lesions are *pathological*, i.e., diseased areas. White matter lesions are associated with stroke. As truth would have it, migraineurs have also been found to be twice as likely to have a stroke as the general population. Even though not all migraineurs have been tested for white matter lesions, I'd be willing to bet if all were tested, all would have white matter lesions, and that their migraines stem from these lesions. But again, the lesions are *caused* by mercury damaging the glutamatergic system allowing glutamates to damage the brain. Where glutamate is excessive, nitric oxide is created to excess (it is trying to come to the rescue) and initiates the firestorm of neurological activity that is a migraine.

What Exactly is Nitric Oxide?

Nitric oxide is a compound in the body (and elsewhere, like in the air) that has both positive and negative actions. Nitric oxide acts as a vasodilator which is intricately involved in migraines (because we know that "swollen" vessels, or *vasodilation*, are part of the "things going on" in migraines). Like so many activities in the body, in the right amounts, nitric oxide does beneficial things, and too little can actually deprive the body of those beneficial things. Conversely, too much nitric oxide is highly toxic — as in migraines. Our understanding of nitric oxide is quite new. It was only in 1998, when the Nobel prize was awarded to Robert F. Furchgott, Ferid Murad and Louis J. Ignarro for their discoveries regarding the various roles of nitric oxide in cardiovascular physiology.

Nitric oxide (NO) is a biological messenger molecule **produced by one of the essential amino acids L-arginine** by the catalytic action of the enzyme NO synthase (NOS). The dual role of NO as a protective or toxic molecule is due to several factors, such as the isoform of NOS involved, concentration of NO and the type of cells in which it is synthesised, the availability of the substrate L-arginine, generation of guanosine 3,5'-cyclic monophosphate (cGMP) from soluble guanylate cyclase and the overall extra and intracellular environment in which NO is produced. **NOS activation as a result of trauma (calcium influx) or infection leads to NO production,** which activates its downstream receptor sGC to synthesise cGMP and/or leads to protein nitrosylation. This may lead to one or more systemic effects including **altered neurotransmission which can be protective or toxic...** [*Histol Histopathol.* 2006 Apr;21(4):445-58.]

Nitric oxide (NO) mediates pathogenic changes in the brain... endogenous NO increases the [Ca(2+)](i) response... an involvement of L-type Ca(2+) channels in the NO-mediated mechanisms... significantly increased by L-arginine...vitamin C decomposes nitrosothiol... reversed the change in the Ca(2+) current with L-arginine....an **elevated endogenous NO production enhances the influx of Ca(2+)** [*Free Radic Biol Med.* 2007 Jan 1;42(1):52-63.]

Before you give up and think that all of this is too difficult to understand, I urge you to stick with it. The most important overall things for you to understand are bulleted at the end of chapter one, and things you can do specifically for migraines are outlined at the end of this chapter. But if you don't at least attempt to understand some of this, you'll be kept in the dark your entire life. Honestly, that would make many of the doctors I've met quite happy. Case in point, one doctor I was talking to said mockingly and under his breath, "Oooh, researching on the internet...*dangerous.*" Funny thing - he never had any answers for me, but the internet had many.

That doctor's fear, of course, was that by my understanding what I had, what has been tried and didn't work, the danger of various drugs, and such, he could not do as he usually did, and simply prescribe drugs or surgery for me. People that "know too much" also ask a lot of questions also take up too much time – and *time is money.* Well, that pretty much left him not knowing *what* to do.

It appears that nitric oxide comes to the rescue after a glutamate-induced neural firestorm. This is because the glutamate-induced neural firestorm causes vessels to constrict, and nitric oxide, wanting to save you from that constriction and the lack of oxygen it would cause, is a vasodilator. The internally-produced nitric oxide also causes an influx of calcium [$Ca(2+)$] into your cells.

Ca2+influx induces chemokine production in monocytes that aggravates **inflammatory** neutrophil infiltration. [*Nat Med* 2008 Jul;14(7):738-47.]

This study above is saying the reverse, that an influx of calcium into your cells is one of the factors that leads to inflammation (caused by nitric oxide and a cascade of events). The influx of calcium is why doctors give heart patients *calcium channel blockers.* Heart disease involves inflammation and could very well also be a result of mercury damage to the glutamatergic system and subsequent excess neural firing as well. Actually, if you string together various studies, what emerges is clear evidence that nitric oxide both increases the influx of calcium into cells and the calcium influx causes an increase in nitric oxide. It's a vicious cycle!

Nitroglycerin Leads To Nitric Oxide Production

One model of migraine headache is the systemic administration of nitric oxide (NO) donor **nitroglycerin** (NTG), which triggers a delayed attack without aura in many migraine patients but not in healthy volunteers... **nitric oxide triggers migraine attacks.** [Varga H et al. The modulatory effect of estrogen on the caudal trigeminal nucleus of the rat in an animal model of migraine *Ideggyogy Sz.* 2006 Nov 20;59(11-12):389-95.]

Nitroglycerin was first discovered in 1847 by Ascanio Sobrero in Turin who was continuing the work of Theophile-Jules Pelouze. Sobrero first noticed that nitroglycerin would induce *violent headaches* even using a very tiny quantity of the substance on the tongue. In 1849 Constantin Hering tested nitroglycerin on healthy volunteers, noting that the headache was reproduced time and again without fail. Nitroglycerin was later officially recognized as a powerful vasodilator (which, of course, is one of the problems in migraine, and why it caused the "violent headache" without fail). In 1867 Lauder Brunton, the father of modern pharmacology, used nitroglycerin to relieve angina. Dilating blood vessels stimulates the oxygenation and flow of blood to the heart and throughout the body. Unfortunately *excess* nitric oxide is very damaging.

Nitric Oxide has been shown to induce cellular injury via inhibition of the mitochondrial respiratory chain and/or oxidative/nitrosative stress. [*Life Sci.* 2006 Sep 20;79(17):1606-15.]

Arginine Leads To Nitric Oxide Production

It is obvious from my own experience as well as the scientific studies that a migraineur produces far too much nitric oxide, which is, of course, in response to a damaged glutamatergic system coupled with the ingestion of factors that stimulate glutamate release – as well as the ingestion of glutamate itself! On the other side of the fence are people with angina, cardiovascular problems, or impotence, producing far too little nitric oxide. Did you know that Viagra is a nitric oxide producer?

The building block of nitric oxide is **arginine**, an amino acid. Arginine is called a "nonessential amino acid" in that it can be manufactured in the body by the assembling of other amino acids. Arginine is intricately involved in the stimulation of cell growth and muscle growth but also the stimulation of aberrant cell growth including cancer and viral overgrowth.

People who harbor herpes (something like 85% of all people do) but especially people who have cancer, as well as migraines, all need to avoid foods that have a greater level of arginine in relation to lysine. Lysine is the "opposing" amino acid to arginine and is known to *block* viral growth. Lysine is the supplement of choice when you feel a cold sore coming on or any other viral outbreak. Foods that are higher in arginine than lysine are nuts, seeds and chocolate and should *never* be consumed by a migraineur. A migraineur would also be wise to limit or eliminate high gluten grains (also high in arginine, but not as high as that found in nuts, seeds and chocolate). The permanent change should be to eliminate glutenous grains, nuts, seeds and chocolate, and instead choose corn, potatoes, yams and rice for starch needs. Go to http://www.herpes.com/Nutrition.shtml (or search for **Ratio of Lysine to Arginine in Certain Foods**, by James M. Scutero) for an extensive chart showing the lysine to arginine ratio. Stick to the foods with a 1.000 or greater ratio for optimizing lysine and minimizing arginine. This doesn't mean you won't get enough arginine for health and proper growth. It *does* mean you will limit the building blocks for nitric oxide excess as well as viral overgrowth. For example, a 200 gram persimmon has 55 mg of lysine and 42 mg of arginine. The ratio is 1.310, i.e., more lysine than arginine. This is a good food for migraineurs.

Persimmon 200 55 42 1.310

One-hundred grams of walnuts contain 466 mg of lysine to 2,520 mg. of arginine, a 0.185 ratio. This is one of the worst foods for migraineurs, as well as people with herpes or cancer.

Walnuts 100 466 2520 0.185

The goal is to *not* fuel nitric oxide!

...Using the glyceryl trinitrate [GTN; **nitric oxide** (NO) donor] model of experimental **headache**... (brain.oxfordjournals.org/cgi/content/abstract/123/9/1830)

Another chemical in the body that may play a role in tension **headache** is **nitric oxide**, which is involved in the transmission of nerve impulses. (www.cnn.com/HEALTH/library/DS/00304.html)

Nitric oxide (NO) can induce **headache** in migraine patients (www.neurotransmitter.net/migraineno.html)

Nitric oxide-induced **headache** may arise from extracerebral arteries as judged from tolerance to isosorbide-5-mononitrate (www.ncbi.nlm.nih.gov/pubmed/18521538)

Glutamates Lead To Nitric Oxide Production

The glutamate sources are both endogenous glutamates (those your body makes internally) and those from the literal tons of free glutamates now put into our processed foods. Some farmers are even spraying free glutamates on their crops! One product used is Auxigro. (See: http://www.truthinlabeling.org/msgsprayed.html)

> High concentrations of **glutamate** can accumulate in the brain and may be involved in the pathogenesis of **neurodegenerative disorders** such as Alzheimer's disease. This form of neurotoxicity involves changes in the regulation of cellular calcium (Ca2+) and generation of free radicals such as peroxynitrite (ONOO-) *i.e., nitric oxide. BMC* [*Neurosci.* 2005 May 10;6(1):34.]

Glutamates are *everywhere.* Food manufacturers *know* they're highly undesirable. Thus, the manufacturers hide them within other ingredients because the FDA has ruled that if glutamates are a *part* of another ingredient, the product doesn't have to list MSG, monosodium glutamate or glutamate as an ingredient. Can you imagine? That's no different than saying if you mix yellow and red paint, making orange, you can lie and say there's no "red" in the mix simply because it now *looks* orange. But what if you're deathly allergic to red? In this case food manufacturers are innocent of any charges if you get migraines, Alzheimer's or even if you die. If I could accomplish something extraordinarily worthwhile to mankind, my desire would be to *completely ban free glutamates from being added to our foods.* Every time I see anyone eating the chemical concoction called "Top Ramen" it's as if I'm watching someone consume poison unknowingly. Note the ingredients of this very popular "soup" (this brand is "Traditional" Ramen noodle soup):

Ingredients
Enriched Wheat Flour (Wheat Flour, Thiamine Mononitrate, Riboflavin, Niacin, Reduced Iron, Folic Acid, Amylase, Benzoyl Peroxide, Ascorbic Acid), Hydrogenated Vegetable Oil (Canola and/or Soy and/or Palm), Salt, **Monosodium Glutamate**, Maltodextrin, Sugar, Dehydrated Vegetables (Onion, Celery, Garlic, Parsley), **Hydrolyzed Soy, Corn & Wheat Protein**, Natural Flavor (**Yeast Extract**, Thiamine Hydrochloride, Partially Hydrogenated Soybean Oil), Canola Oil, Dextrose Monohydrate, Spice and Coloring, Calcium Silicate (Anticaking Agent), Potassium Carbonate, Sodium Tripolyphosphate, Guar Gum, Spices, Disodium Inosinate, Disodium Guanylate,

Sodium Carbonate, Fd&c Yellow No. 5 Lake, **Spice Extractives**, BHA & BHT (Antioxidants).

All of the ingredients above emphasized in **bold** contain free glutamates, and of course monosodium gluatamte is 100% pure "free glutamates". It's rare that a manufacturer will blatantly put in pure MSG. But there it is. Overall, the ingredients read like a toxic dump, not food. "Spice Extractives" is also usually a free glutamate source – that's why they don't tell you which spices, and is yet another way the FDA allows glutamates to be hidden. Our laws require that food ingredients be listed in order of amount. So the first ingredient is the one that exists in the greatest quantity and on down until you get to the last ingredient, which exists in the least quantity in the food. Note how on the above list pure monosodium glutamate is the fourth ingredient, even before vegetables! Very frightening.

Monosodium glutamate was first used in the US in the late 1940s. By the 1960s, Accent, the leading brand of the flavor enhancer called "monosodium glutamate," had become a household word. Simultaneously, other **hydrolyzed protein** products such as **autolyzed yeast, sodium caseinate**, and **hydrolyzed vegetable protein** gained in popularity. Every hydrolyzed* protein product, regardless of the name given to it on a label, contains MSG. (*also all isolated, fermented, texturized protein products) [From "Ask Yahoo" http://answers.yahoo.com]

Where Else Do "Free Glutamates" Come From?

When I became a "health foodist" due to my attempts to get rid of my psoriasis from about age 11 on, I consumed copious quantities of "health foods". I don't mean whole, organic fruits and vegetables, I mean "Dr. Jensen's Seasoning Broth", Bragg liquid aminos, fermented and hydrolyzed soy products, etc. If only I'd known then what I know now. These foods are all toxic sources of *free glutamates.* When you modify, hydrolyze, isolate, ferment or otherwise alter proteins (e.g., by adding enzymes), you generate free glutamates (as well as other free amino acids).

> All **processed soy products** — soy milk, soy burgers, soy cheese, soy energy bars, soy ice cream, soy protein powders, etc. — are <u>not</u> health foods. And to truly avoid all types of damaging soy products, you need to avoid processed foods as the vast majority of them contain soy ingredients. "The best — and maybe the only — way to completely avoid soy in the food supply is to buy whole foods and prepare them ourselves," [Kaayla T. Daniel, PhD]
>
> Soy might be hiding in ingredient lists, look for words like "bouillon," "natural flavor" and "textured plant protein."

You can read the entire article by Dr. Mercola regarding Dr. Daniel's book at: http://articles.mercola.com/sites/articles/archive/2008/09/16/what-s-so-bad-about-tofu.aspx. Dr. Daniel talks about soy as being high in "natural toxins". Getting back to looking at everything from God's point of view, this is not at all surprising. We're not meant to "fool around" with foods in their natural state. Yet soy is most often highly processed to make many protein-altered products. During the processing, nutrients are destroyed, altered, mutated, and more. The result is the generation of what Dr. Daniel calls "antinutrients" or substances that work *against* your health.

Antinutrients include various "inhibitors", which are substances you consume when you consume the altered food products. These inhibitors keep enzymes from digesting and doing what enzymes are designed to do. This can cause distress throughout the gastro-intestinal tract of which you aren't even aware. If you already have a defective immune system, damaged by mercury and other pollutants, like pesticides (which soy products are notoriously excessively high in!) you can exacerbate your "leaky gut" syndrome. (Review Chapter 4 *Parasites* section on fungus). Of course leaky gut syndrome leads to many ailments including skin diseases, allergies and more.

Dr. Daniel also talks about fermented, isolated, hydrolyzed, etc. soy products being high in substances that cause hemagglutination. This means altered soy puts foreign molecules into the blood which cause red blood cells to clump together. Soy proteins contain goitrogens which can lead to depressed thyroid function. I don't see where Dr. Daniel discusses how the fermentation and processing of soy generates extremely high levels of free glutamates. But it does during the extensive process of fermentation, isolation, and hydrolyzation, as this is when the amino acid glutamate is cleaved from what it is bonded to, to generate "free" glutamates. Again, these are not found in Nature. Yet many of our most intelligent people believe that "glutamates" are natural. Indeed they are, but only if bonded to others things as found in nature. Another "natural" substance is arsenic, but not when extracted and sprinkled on your food! Both are "found" in nature. Neither are meant for humans to collect, concentrate and consume.

Your Body Makes All The Glutamate It Needs For Neural Synapsing

Indeed, your own body generates all the glutamate it needs for the infintisimal amount required to cause neurons to fire, synapse (connect) and thus do their work in your brain and central nervous system. Any free glutamates you ingest are in excess of what is needed. The *tons* of free glutamates being added to our foods on a daily basis is frightening - moreso than you realize. If people truly knew the damage glutamates are causing, and glutamate's contribution to neurological diseases, aging, pain, and just about every health problem - they would instantly refuse to purchase anything containing them. Yet every time a consumer purchases a packaged or seasoned food, it is *most* likely to contain free glutamates (or another common excitotoxin, aspartate).

Go to www.truthinlabeling.org to get the list of glutamate sources. As you read this list, keep in mind that if they say it "may" be a source of glutamate, you need to assume that it *is* a source. For example, parmesan cheese doesn't list a glutamate source on its label, but lists "enzymes" added, and these enzymes *generate* glutamates (enzymes act upon the protein to free the glutamate). I know because the purpose of those enzymes is to alter the proteins, *and* because my ability to handle even a molecule of glutamate is completely destroyed and consuming parmesan gives me a migraine every time.

Unbeknownst to you, the foods you consume on a daily basis if they have seasonings and other additivies - even if found in a "health food store", are *full* of excitotoxins. Excitotoxins are amino acids that food manufacturers add to your food to "excite" your tastebuds. In this way, inferior foods taste superior. But glutamates and other excitotoxins (like aspartate as in "Aspartame") go to your brain and central nervous system and *damage your brain and central nervous system.*

A Cure For Migraines

Why one person will have chronic migraines and another have them only periodically; or why one person has them for years and years, and another person suddenly stops having them, has to do with how badly damaged the glutamatergic system is, whether or not they have estrogen peaks, whether or not they consume free glutamates, how bad their white matter lesions are, etc. At this time, the only way I can see for migraines to be "cured" would be to stop the damaging elements (mercury and glutamates), and then have neural stem cells injected directly into the area of the brain that has been damaged.

Objective: To investigate a possibility of **repairing damaged brain** by intracerebroventricular transplantation of neural stem cells (NSCs) in the adult mice subjected to **glutamate-induced excitotoxic injury.** Results: Intracerebroventricular **transplantation of neural stem cells** may be feasible in repairing diseased or damaged brain tissue. [Ma J et al. Repair of glutamate-induced excitotoxic neuronal damage mediated by intracerebroventricular transplantation of neural stem cells in adult mice. *Neurosci Bull* 2007 Jul;23(4):209-14.]

Genuine Healing – Regenerative Medicine

CBS – Cutting Edge, March 23, 2008. Lee Spievack sliced off the tip of his finger in a hobby shop accident. Spievack's brother Alan, sent him a special powder to sprinkle on the wound. Every bit of Lee's finger grew back – the flesh, the blood vessels, the nails, everything – in four weeks. Dr. Steven Badylak of the University of Pittsburgh's McGowan Institute of Regenerative Medicine said the powder was made from pig bladders called "extracellular matrix". It's a mixture of protein and connective tissue that surgeons often use to repair tendons. Scientists who are using it say that every tissue in the body has cells capable of complete regeneration. The matrix summons those cells and tells them what to do. This is an arm of medicine called Regenerative Medicine.

In his lab at Wake Forest University, a lab he calls a medical factory, Dr. Anthony Atala and co-workers are growing body parts, among them, 18-different types of muscles tissue and heart valves. They are making body parts to plant right back into patients. Dr. Atala also believes that every type of tissue has cells ready to regenerate if only researchers do the right things to prod them into action. They grew the heart of a mouse by spraying heart mouse stem cells into the pattern of a heart. Cells have all the information necessary to make new tissue. Everybody's heart has cells programmed and ready to make more heart cells. This applies also to your bladder, your kidney and every other tissue. They use the patients own cells, increasing the cells in the lab. The cells differentiate into the various cells that make up the tissue. Is this the future? The scientists say yes, but they also say, it's *today*. The video below says that the U.S. Army Institute of Surgical Research has invested millions in this type of regenerative therapy. Go to: http://www.youtube.com/watch?v=qxhi4Q8EDTU or in Google, type in: CBS – Cutting Edge, March 23, 2008.

It is clear to me as it should be to you. Regenerative medicine needs to be our *first* line of medicine, not something we "try" when the flawed methods we are currently using fail to work. Unfortunately what is currently happening in medicine is an urgency to "attack" a disease with radiation, chemicals and surgery. Not only does this fail to assist the body's own mechanisms of healing and regeneration, but the burning, poisoning and cutting out of cells and tissues *greatly interferes if not completely stops* a patient's own regenerative powers. This has *got* to stop! People go in for cancer therapies, and within a few months to a few years, most are dead – but after much suffering. Any that survive are so drained financially, emotionally and physically, even if they had access to regenerative medicine, they wouldn't be able to use it.

Stem cells need to become available and affordable as soon as possible! The problems are political and greed. The so-called debate continues to rage about stem cells (mostly over the ethics of using embryonic) while benevolent scientists are quietly doing their research using bone marrow and umbilical cord stem cells, and/or are forced by law to do their research mostly on animals. The "debate" is really a monetary issue, as scientists paid by drug companies strive for the big bucks by holding out for using only embryonic stem cells because it is a source they can predictably produce and thus patent. Meanwhile umbilical cord stem cells and even your own stem cells are ready and available now for use! For more information call The Steenblock Research Institute (800) 288-7016. Or visit: http://www.stemcelltherapies.org/ They can help you get on a path of learning more about various types of stem cell therapies currently available, as well as what's in the works for future use.

Infection (Viral, Bacterial, Fungal) Leads To Excess Nitric Oxide Production

George E. Meinig, DDS wrote the book called "Root Canal Coverup Exposed" in which he brings to our attention the massive work of Dr. Weston Price. Dr. Price led a team of some 60 scientists and physicians who found that root canaled teeth contain about 3 miles of microscopic canals within the dentin of the dead teeth that harbor deadly bacteria. These bacteria mutate into highly toxic anaerobic organisms as deadly as botulism that travel throughout the body and set up infections wherever they go. Dr. Price is responsible for proving *the focal infection theory*. In extensive research, he took root canaled teeth out of very ill people and implanted them just under the skin of rabbits. He did this hundreds of times and the rabbits *without fail* would get the exact same disease the person had!

Dr. Meinig points out that someone with a super strong immune system will fight these deadly bacteria and may never show the effects of the invasion, or may only succumb after some other event weakens their immune system, like surgery, or having an amalgam filling placed. But people who have damaged immune systems already, such as migraineurs whose DNA, mitochondria, glutamatergic system, and entire immune system has been damaged by mercury from amalgams, eating fish, flu shots (and other immunizations) *cannot* handle the deadly bacteria which migrate to diseased tissues, such as the areas in the brain or central nervous sytem that have been damaged. Below we see how anaerobic bacteria generate nitric oxide. Nitrate (NO3) is the primary source of nitrogen (N) for plants and is a nutrient they cannot live without. Even if you consume a natural diet, water and food supplies nitrate. Processed meats contain nitrite.

We conclude that **nitric oxide** can be **generated by the anaerobic gut flora** in the presence of nitrate or nitrite. [**Sobko T** et al. Gastrointestinal bacteria generate nitric oxide from nitrate and nitrite. Nitric Oxide. 2005 Dec;13(4):272-8.]

Dr. Meinig told Dr. Mercola in an interview:

"My book is based upon Dr. Weston Price's twenty-five years of careful, impeccable research. He led a 60-man team of researchers whose findings (suppressed until now) rank right up there with the greatest medical discoveries of all time. This is not the usual medical story of a prolonged search for the difficult-to-find causative agent of some devastating disease. Rather, it's the story of how a "cast of millions" (i.e., bacteria) become entrenched inside the structure of teeth and end up causing the largest number of diseases ever traced to a single source."

So bacteria contribute mightily to migraines because in the end they stimulate the production of excess nitric oxide. Just like continuously, internally-produced estrogen, the internally-produced bacteria produce continuous fuel for the production of nitric oxide. This is well beyond a damaged immune and glutamatergic system's ability to cope. But *unlike* estrogen, the bacteria from a root canaled tooth is 24/7, 365 days a year (your entire life) until you *remove* the source, i.e., the dead, root canaled tooth (or teeth). In fact root canals and other rotting teeth can be a continuous source of nitric oxide stimuli that cause your *worst* and frequent migraines.

I say it elsewhere, and it bears repeating perhaps more than anything else in this book: After having my 3 root canals removed, my migraines virtually *disappeared.* (See Chapter 6 *Dental Work*). I bought and read the book in the textbox below, months after having my own root canals out. But what Dr. Huggins and Dr. Levy say is *exactly* what has happened to me. It doesn't mean I don't have to continue taking supplements against nitric oxide, or that I can stop completely avoiding glutamates. It *does* mean, while doing all the right things, I am now enjoying far fewer and far less painful migraines!

Talking about after the removal of root canals, mercury, and other sources of toxins in the mouth: "People with migraines will experience a reduction in both number and intensity, such that they do not have to take prescription drugs, and are not debilitated. Over-the-counter drugs will handle the new level. There are some people who will move from migraines to no headaches at all..." [Hal A. Huggins DDS MS and Thomas E Levy MD, JD *Uninformed Consent The Hidden Dangers In Dental Care.*]

The bottom-line truth remains, *mercury* is the culprit that caused you to become a migraineur. Had you never been exposed to mercury, you would *not* have migraines. The devastating effects of the mercury's damage to your cell's structure, including the DNA and mitochondria, include a glutamatergic system gone berserk. That out-of-control glutamatergic system cannot handle the various "agents" that ignite it's neural activity. These agents *include* bacteria, but also free glutamates, nitric oxide itself (e.g., if you take nitroglycerin), estrogen rise and fall, and various visual and olfactory stimuli. In the end, migraines are all about the excessive stimulation of neurons, and the inability of your body to stop those neurons from firing excessively.

Migraines and the Military

In August, 2008, the headline read: Army Personnel Show Increased Risk For Migraine; Condition Underdiagnosed, Mistreated.

> The findings show that 19 percent of **soldiers** returning from Iraq screened positive for **migraine** and an additional 17 percent screened positive for possible migraine. Soldiers with a positive migraine screen suffered a mean average of 3.1 headache days per month. [*Science Daily* Aug. 28, 2008]

The article goes on to say that military personnel are likely to encounter various physiological and psychological factors that are "known" to precipitate migraine attacks. The factors they list are disrupted sleep and meal patterns, fatigue, psychological stress, emotional strain, heat, noise and other environmental exposures (*all* of which stimulate excessive neural activity, by the way, leading to elevated nitric oxide). Blaming migraines on anything and everything is common and it's because those doing the blaming have absolutely no clue what *caused* a person to get migraines in the first place, and what *initiates* each neurological firestorm in the second place.

I bring this up because nowhere in the article is mercury, thimerosal, neurons behaving badly, or glutamates, mentioned, yet they are among the most important causal factors. To merely mention the "stimuli" is like stating the obvious. All migraineurs know that a day at Disneyland might precipitate a migraine. We need to know *why* it does. The real truth is that military personnel are subject both to a higher amount of immunizations (**mercury**) that are forced upon them as well as **free glutamates** in their typically processed foods diet. And the fact is that stimuli wouldn't stimulate a migraine if there'd been no mercury or glutamate damage in the first place. Additionally, so-called stimuli can be drastically lessened and even stopped if *free glutamates* are taken completely out of the diet.

In another report called "Immunizations For Military Trainees" by Renata Engler, M.D. and others, a table shows that military in the American Revolutionary War, 1775-1783 and through the Spanish-American War, 1898, only received a single smallpox vaccine (and thimerosal hadn't been conceived yet). Then during World War II the number of immunizations sky-rocketed to 12 vaccines. World War II was in 1941-1945, so that these vaccines would have contained thimerosal most likely, since the mercury-containing "preservative" was created in 1930. In 2001 and today military personnel receive 15 different vaccines with several more being planned. I'm told by one marine that some vaccines he received have been from "multiuse" vials (very likely contain mercury), but that a recent flu vaccine was delivered by nasal-mist, which my information shows does not contain mercury.

Considering that *no amount of mercury* is safe, if any of these 15 vaccines contain mercury, for military personnel who have already had their share of immunizations as children, and if they also have amalgam fillings (I believe the military dentists also currently only use amalgam for fillings), its easy to see why the incidence of migraine would be high in this population. Sadly, the incidence of Lou Gehrig's, perhaps the most devastating of all neurological diseases, is *also* prevalent in this population.

Actually, the statistics for migraines is high in the general population as well! Some statistics say that 25% of women and 8% of men get migraines sometime in their lifetime. If you use these statistics, that's 1 in 4 women! For men it amounts to 8 out of every 100 men. I'm not sure how reliable *any* statistics are. But in the case of migraine statistics, I know that I wouldn't be included because I don't go to doctors for my migraines – and mine have been among the worst migraines a person could have (i.e., chronic and severe). So, how many other people aren't included in the statistics? Then you'd have to ask, how many are included, but are having "headaches" and not migraines? The important thing is that migraines are far too common, and everybody knows somebody that gets them. That's enough of an epidemic for me!

There's No Question that 1 in 4 Gulf War Veterans Suffers From Illness Caused by Exposure to Pesticides and Other Neurotoxic Chemicals - Research Panel Reports. They list excess toxic exposure to many agents which include: 1) the drug pyridostigmine bromide 2) pesticides 3) exposure to nerve agents and smoke from burning oil wells 4) *receipt of a large number of vaccines* and 5) troops being downwind from the Khamisiyah demolitions

They say that Gulf War Veterans have a much **higher rate of ALS** (Lou Gehrig's Disease) than any other veterans [by Boston University School of Public Health, November 17, 2008]

Estrogen Drop Causes An Excess Nitric Oxide Production

Some other factors can initiate what ends in excess nitric oxide production and thus a neurological firestorm in the damaged brain (thus a migraine in a migraneur or tremors in someone with Parkinson's). Some are: Sudden drop in blood sugar, caffeine withdrawal, adrenalin, drop or fluctuations in estrogen and consumption of high arginine foods (which includes all nuts, seeds, chocolate and grains).

Estrogens fluctuations, particularly their **premenstrual fall**, are currently regarded as the main triggers of menstrual migraine... [Allais G et al. Menstrual migraine: clinical and therapeutical aspects. *Expert Rev Neurother.* 2007 Sep;7(9):1105-20.]

In addition, your eyes and nostrils are hotbeds of neural activity, and excess stimuli to vision or smell can also lead to elevated nitric oxide and a migraine.

Female migraineurs are all too well aware that estrogen is one of the "factors" ultimately leading to a migraine. But doctors don't tell you (because they probably don't know) that a drop in estrogen sparks neurotransmitter activity (glutamates) which leads to the elevated nitric oxide levels that cause the migraine.

Biochemical and genetic evidence suggest central and peripheral roles for **estrogen** in the pathophysiology of menstrual migraine, with potential **interactions with excitatory circuits**...[Brandes JL. The influence of estrogen on migraine: a systematic review. *JAMA*. 2006 Apr 19;295(15):1824-30.]

The reason "menstrual migraines" are so brutal, is because the source of the problem is a continuous supply within the body – it's not something you can simply "turn off".

...a **delay in recovery of the glutamatergic system** along with decreased tone of inhibitory neurotransmitter systems could make the late luteal and early follicular phases of the menstrual cycle (eg, **perimenstrual time**) a particularly vulnerable time for **migraine** headache... During the late luteal and early follicular phases, there is up-regulation of the sympathetic system... [http://www.medscape.com/viewarticle/522000_8]

This is why giving estrogen as a therapy is ultimately disastrous for a migraineur who cannot handle the hormone properly. "The bigger the rise, the greater the fall" proves out in women who are given estrogen in an attempt to cure their migraines. Researchers in 2000 discovered that it's the "drop" that does the dirty deed, so there is no amount of giving estrogen or taking it away that solves the problem. Why? Because *mercury damage to the glutamatergic system* is the true underlying *cause*.

Menstrually-related migraine (MM) appears to be the **withdrawal of estrogen** rather than the maintenance of sustained high or low estrogen levels. Hormonal replacement with estrogens can exacerbate migraine and oral contraceptives (OCs) can change its character and frequency. [Silverstein SD Sex hormones and headache. *Rev Neurol* (Paris) 2000]

It also doesn't help to give progesterone, because progesterone can be converted in the body to estrogen, especially in someone with a damaged system.

> Natural **progesterone** is also different from estrogen in that your body can use it as a precursor or starting material to make other hormones such as adrenal hormones. It can even **convert it into estrogen** or testosterone if your body needs it. [http://www.mercola.com/article/progesterone/cream.htm]

Many woman have experienced their *first* migraine after starting hormone replacement therapy – and it's a whopper! The answer to the hormone question is to allow the body all the time it needs to figure out that menopause is coming, and the body will adjust if given the proper nutrition. What doctors don't tell women is that when the ovary supply of estrogen becomes insufficient, the adrenals will take over – *if given the chance!* Millions of women worldwide have never used hormone replacement therapy and lived long, healthy lives.

> …**female sex steroids** (i.e., **estrogens**) have been shown to enhance: (i) **neuronal excitability** by elevating $Ca(2+)$ and decreasing $Mg(2+)$ concentrations, an action that may occur with other mechanisms triggering migraine; (ii) **the synthesis and release of nitric oxide (NO)** and neuropeptides, such as **calcitonin gene-related peptide CGRP**, a mechanism that reinforces **vasodilatation** and activates trigeminal sensory afferents with a subsequent stimulation of pain centres; and (iii) the function of receptors mediating vasodilatation, while the responses of receptors inducing vasoconstriction are attenuated. The serotonergic, adrenergic and gamma-aminobutyric acid (GABA)-ergic systems are also modulated by sex steroids, albeit to a varying degree and with potentially contrasting effects on migraine outcome. [Gupta S et al. Potential role of female sex hormones in the pathophysiology of migraine. *Pharmacol Ther* 2007 Feb;113(2):321-40.]

In fact, just a few years ago a major proclamation came over the TV and radio airways: *Hormone replacement therapy is dangerous for* every *woman and* will *lead to cancer.* They went so far as to say in "four out of four women" hormone replacement therapy will lead to a cancer of some type. As quickly as that proclamation was made, it "disappeared" into the drug industries secret hiding place where they keep truths that could lose them millions or even billions in profits.

This study below says what I said above — *giving estrogen during a woman's cycle* could prove disastrous (lead to a migraine) by delaying the recovery of the glutamatergic system.

> ...the risk for migraine headache varies during different phases of the menstrual cycle based on a delicate balance of neurotransmitter systems. **Increasing serum levels of estrogen during the mid-cycle** could enhance neurotransmission in the TNC by **enhancing glutamatergic tone** and **predispose to mid-cycle migraine headaches**...a **delay in recovery of the glutamatergic system** along with decreased tone of inhibitory neurotransmitter systems could make the late luteal and early follicular phases of the menstrual cycle (eg, perimenstrual time) a particularly vulnerable time for migraine headache. [Vincent T. Martin MD, Michael Behbehani PhD (2006) Ovarian Hormones and Migraine Headache: Understanding Mechanisms and Pathogenesis—Part I Volume 46 Issue I Page 3-23, January 2006]

There are *no* safe drugs to stop this natural process. The mercury damaged area of the brain and the damage that has been done to the glutamatergic system make estrogen fluctuations your worst enemy. The best that can be done is to help "calm the neurological firestorm" by not feeding the fire. The many ways you can do that are explained in Chapter 11 *Nature's Medicines.* You can go from migraines so horrific you are rushed to the emergency room, to migraines so mild all you need is an Excedrin or two and you're back to work. You just have to get all your "ducks in a row" (right diet, right dentistry, right supplements, avoiding the toxic substances, etc.)

Dangerous Drugs

Unfortunately pain medications given to alleviate migraines are very dangerous. If you don't know that Imitrex or Frova or another anti-migraine drug is what has led to your joint pain, disc degeneration, immune problems, etc., you need to educate yourself before you give in to other dangerous drugs or even surgery.

Triptans

When I tried the "triptans" for just three months I ended up with lupus-like symptoms: A red butterfly rash across my nose, severe joint pain, depression and severe breathing problems. After stopping the medication, it took over a year to dissipate. Perhaps you have these symptoms and just think you're falling apart, not connecting the drugs you take with worsening health. Don't be a victim of thinking these horrific symptoms are an entirely unrelated course of events, and not related to the medications. *They are **caused** by them.* Stop them immediately and start doing the things you need to do to minimize the severity and regularity with which you get migraines. It *can* be done.

The way triptans work is by stopping the activity of CGRP and possibly nitric oxide as well. What is CGRP? Calcitonin gene-related peptide (a protein molecule made up of two or more amino acids – the building blocks of protein). CGRP is part of the "inflammatory pathway" and is the molecule, along with nitric oxide, that causes *vasodilitation*. CGRP is thought to be the molecule involved in *pain transmission*. The higher the level of CGRP, the more pain will be felt. Unfortunately, like all natural processes in the body, CGRP is involved in the physiological functioning of all major systems in the body, respiratory, endocrine, gastrointestinal, immune and cardiovascular. So some degree of vasodilatation is absolutely essential or you have ischemia (lack of blood flow to an area). If you give a drug to stop CGRP and nitric oxide dead in their tracks, you can do as much harm as good!

So triptans are drugs that stop CGRP and nitric oxide, stopping vasodilatation which in turn stops the inflammation and pain. For most migraineurs the migraine stops very quickly. Unfortunately drugs don't know to behave themselves and just stop CGRP in the brain and not go anywhere else. Triptans, like all drugs, go throughout the body. People have had major heart-related complications, including death. But most people taking the drug will be damaged over time, never connecting the drug with their damage. Unfortunately the body also soon begins to rely on the drug to shrink the swollen vasculature, requiring more and more of the drug, which becomes ever more dangerous and toxic.

Bahman Guyuron, MD of Case Western Reserve University Medical Center says that in a migraine you have both vasoconstriction and vasodilatation going on at the same time. Triptans will constrict overly dilated and painful vessels which will relieve the pain of a migraine, but simultaneously and *dangerously* constrict the already constricted vessels that is the second half of a migraine. This can lead to heart complications, and ischemia (like strokes) in various parts of the body leading to damage and disease – especially when taken on a long-term basis.

Get To The Core Of The Problem

You can't just take dangerous drugs to address a problem that at its core involves damage and ongoing assault by offending chemicals. You can't, that is, if you wish to avoid worse complications like a stroke – not to mention, never really getting rid of your migraines in the first place!

Of course eliminating all free glutamates (all excitotoxins) from your diet is the very first thing you absolutely *must* do. Do you put bottled salad dressing on your salad at a restaurant? All the commercial ones are full of free glutamates with rare exceptions. Do you choose the soup on the menu? Unless it's homemade with only herbs and plain salt and pepper for seasoning, there are nearly always free glutamates in there. In my favorite salad-bar restaurant free glutamates are in the "vegetarian soup base" they now put in all their soups! (Ask to see the ingredients. The glutamates are hidden in the hydrolyzed and autolyzed yeast, for example.)

I don't pretend to know it all...but unfortunately, most doctors know even less about what *causes* migraines. The truth is there are many natural things that you can do to lessen the production of excess nitric oxide. As proof your doctor knows less, if he had a clue, he would have insisted that the first thing you do is educate yourself about the 40+ excitotoxin food additives, and about the dietary measures you can take to stop excess nitric oxide, instead of writing you out a very dangerous prescription to merely alleviate the pain.

Why You *Can't* Take Unlimited Analgesics

First let's start with why you'd want to take analgesics: Pain. I met a man once when I was doing nutrition consults, who told me he took eight Advil every day. His pain had risen beyond his concern over taking too much of any drug. Even when I told him about "analgesic nephropathy" (destruction of the kidneys from analgesic use) he said he planned to continue to take the Advil. While I completely empathize with pain so bad you wish you could die, I also know that there are God-given means to counteract pain. Counteracting pain begins with understanding why you have the pain.

The pain in diseases of all kinds is caused by inflammation. Inflammation is actually a *disease process.* The end result of redness, heat, and pain *starts* with an immune system that cannot counteract an assault. The assault ultimately, is "oxidative stress". I say ultimately, because it may start with a toxin, like mercury, but in the end, the toxic action is via tremendous oxidative stress. Oxidative stress is the real reason why high cholesterol is "bad", eating fried foods is bad, not getting enough antioxidants is "bad", getting a sunburn is "bad" etc.

The first goal would be to keep the immune system intact (no toxic metals, a super nutrient-dense diet, etc.) *or* to heavily support an already damaged immune system. Indeed, the main reason the immune system would fail to handle oxidative assault is because it has been damaged. Part of your highly complex "immune system" consists of powerful antioxidants in the "sulfur" category that gobble up toxins, deactivate toxins, stand guard at your cells to defend you against toxins – you get the picture. Three of these are alpha-lipoic acid (ALA),

185

glutathione (GSH) and N-acetylcysteine (NAC). As you inhale, slather on, inject or eat any toxin from mercury to acetaminophen (Tylenol), these sulfur-based antioxidants help protect your liver, your kidneys, all your body's cells, from toxic damaging effects.

So here's the bottom line with regard to over-the-counter analgesics: If you take acetaminophen (as in Tylenol or Excedrin) day after day (but this applies to ingesting any toxic substance) your body's ability to fight off the toxic effects *(especially when its already immune-compromised from mercury damage)* becomes more and more impaired – even to the point of organ failure. The two organs that fail most often are the liver and kidneys. Hence, the epidemic of people today on kidney dialysis. You see a new dialysis center on nearly every major city corner these days. Currently there are over 60,000 people on the donor waiting list, and only about 9,000 cadaver kidneys available annually. Many people will die of kidney failure before ever getting a kidney. Others who go on dialysis three days per week quickly become weary of the needles and the long hours the procedure takes. But the kidneys don't just "clean the blood" they also produce important hormones like erythropoietin, a hormone that acts upon stem cells to produce more red blood cells. Yes, with kidney failure comes many problems.

A teenage girl was rushed to the hospital after taking *eight* extra-strength Tylenol in a 12 hour period for pain she couldn't get rid of. Her liver failed and she needed a transplant immediately. Of course that's the extreme side of the story. But unfortunately it's not as rare as it should be. There are teens who binge drink (alcohol uses up the glutathione that protects the liver from toxins), go home with a headache, take a Tylenol, and are found dead in their beds in the morning. Then there are those people who take Tylenol and other analgesics "according to directions". The directions at some point in time were two in a 24-hour period. Now I've noticed manufacturers have gone back to saying four tablets in a 24-hour period are the limit. But studies show that even low doses over long periods of time can cause kidney failure.

I try to save the Excedrin only for migraines. When I have other pain I try to use other methods of coping (see information about T.E.N.S. unit in Chapter 10 *And More* in the "Hip Pain" section).

The Most Important Things You Can Do

By doing all the right things it is possible to drop from one or two horrific migraines per week to only one mild migraine per month or even less. You can improve from migraines that used to send you to bed for an entire day or even three days, to where they don't stop you at all. You can progress from where only dangerous drugs worked, to where over-the-counter analgesics get you back up and running. A pain level of 10+ can drop down to 2 or 3 in severity and you can feel far more in control. You can go from having migraines with nausea and vomiting to possibly never experiencing nausea and vomiting again. You can plan your life around what you want to *do* instead of fearing your plans will be ruined by a migraine.

Of course the even greater goal is to *eliminate* migraines 100%, if not in your life, at least for future generations. I believe this is entirely possible (and only possible when you know what caused them in the first place) if we, once and for all, rid the environment of mercury (and other toxic metals) and of "free glutamates". My prayer is that with this awareness we can do just that. Your dollars speak volumes. *Refuse* to purchase anything that makes use of mercury (find alternatives for these things, or do without) and anything that contains added free glutamates. Below are the five steps you need to implement immediately.

<u>First</u> – Stop all free glutamate sources as well as aspartates. Stop alcohol as it contains altered amino acids generated in the fermentation process as well. Altered proteins are toxic because they stimulate excess nitric oxide and is one of the reasons people with *low* nitric oxide production seem to benefit by alcohol. The beneficial antioxidant resveratrol in wine is also a known stimulator of nitric oxide (good for the heart, bad for the migraine):

> Resveratrol induced a sustained increase in estrogen receptor-dependent **nitric oxide production.** [*J Cardiovasc Pharmacol.* 2007 Jul;50(1):83-93.]

Neither alcohol or glutamates have immediate effects necessarily, which is why most people don't make the connection. In a brain with a damaged glutamatergic system, the toxic proteins set into motion that cascade of events that ends in excessive nitric oxide. That cascade of events can take minutes to a day or more. You *must* be strict about no free glutamates, aspartates or alcohol if you want to eliminate your migraines. If you've ever experienced a hangover, or know of someone who has, they are very similar to a migraine, caused by nitric oxide excess, complete with nausea and vomiting.

Second – Find a dentist that safely removes mercury *and* who knows how to properly extract teeth when needed. Take the list of "Dental Musts" in Chapter 6 with you and interview a potential dentist long before you have an emergency, like a crown popping off. You can also ask people you trust for a recommendation of a holistic dentist. Chronic infection in cavitations, under crowns and in the miles of tubules in root canals is a continuous stimuli for your worst migraines.

Third – Absolutely no more flu shots, vaccinations, or eating fish – *all likely have mercury.* Be aware of all mercury sources and eliminate them, as well as other toxic substances. Do your homework. The internet is a wealth of information. Start by Googling "Mercury, Wikipedia" and read the article there. You'll find that mercury is being spewed into the environment. Again, we must "vote" with our dollars and absolutely refuse to purchase anything with mercury, including those new lightbulbs and long fluorescent bulbs, as they contain mercury. If you find you work where they are used, or for any reason have to use them, if you break one, *do not* simply vacuum or wipe up the mess as the mercury dissipates instantly into the air. Make sure you're not buying into anything with lead, arsenic, cadmium or nickel, as well. You can do something *now* by refusing to purchase anything made using these poisons. Google: "Buy non-toxic" and peruse the websites. Don't wait for the government to protect you – your government is made up of fallible humans, and if something doesn't directly impact their lives, they aren't motivated to do anything.

Fourth You must immediately start to consume a diet that consists of mostly plant foods that are pure, whole (without chemical additives and glutamates) and preferably organic (no pesticides). You need to consume as many raw as possible. The diet needs to favor lysine-rich foods, while avoiding arginine-rich foods. Arginine-rich foods are nuts, seeds, chocolate, but also glutenous grains (wheat, oats, rye, barley). Remember, arginine is the direct building-block of nitric oxide. The best diet would consist of all pure, whole, fresh, (preferably organic), vegetables, beans, fruits, poultry, eggs, with yams, potatoes, corn and rice as your starches.

Fifth Supplements need to emphasize opposing nitric oxide production which includes natural anti-infectives and anti-inflammatories (nitric oxide is part of the infection and inflammation process). (See Chapter 11 *Nature's Medicines*). With migraines, the goal is to stop the ultimate production of nitric oxide in the first place. So eliminating nuts, seeds, chocolate and even grains is crucial (all super high in arginine, nitric oxide's building block). Likely, the most powerful "anti-nitric oxide" supplement that exists is ginger. The heavy use of ginger is actually quite common in some cultures. You can take 2-4 capsules with every meal, or even just your last meal of the day to help keep nitric oxide from building up overnight. Ginger won't "erase" excessive consumption of high arginine foods. However, it may be just the miracle you need on what should be your worst migraine day, i.e., "menstrual" migraine day (although these actually occur postmenopausally as well with the rise and fall of hormones).

Chapter 9
MULTIPLE SCLEROSIS

After reading, you should understand that if you'd never been damaged by **mercury**, you would not have multiple sclerosis; and how mercury and *not* aluminum, lead, cadmium, etc. was proven to **destroy neurons** on contact; that the ability of the body to link **tubulin molecules** together to form the neurite membrane that makes the protective coating around neurons is destroyed by mercury; and thus how "all hell breaks loose" in a brain and body damaged by mercury leading to any of dozens of devastating neurological disorders. "All the things going on" in each person and each neurological disease differs according to where the damage occurs, how many protective systems are in place and working (antioxidants, glutamatergic system, etc.), how much damage you were already born with, how much mercury you've encountered, and how many other toxins you are bombarded with daily (like free glutamates).

There is absolutely *no question* that the pollutant (the "rabbit") that causes multiple sclerosis is **mercury.**

Exogenous toxins, such as **mercury** and other environmental contaminants, exacerbate **mitochondrial electron leakage, hastening their demise** and that of their host cells. Studies of the brain in Alzheimer's and other dementias, Down syndrome, stroke, Parkinson's disease, **multiple sclerosis**, amyotrophic lateral sclerosis, Huntington's disease, Friedreich's ataxia, aging, and constitutive disorders demonstrate impairments of the mitochondrial citric acid cycle and oxidative phosphorylation (OXPHOS) enzymes. [Kidd PM, *Altern Med Rev* 2005 Dec;10(4):268-93.]

Mercury From Hep B Shots

In fact, while pouring over scientific studies to write yet another paper for a doctor, I ran into an article that mentioned how "common" it is for someone to develop multiple sclerosis (MS) after a hepatitis B shot (hepatitis B shots have contained a whopping 12.5 mcg of mercury!) The two articles in the textbox below, don't mention the 12.5 mcg of mercury in the hepatitis B vaccine, and only blame the vaccine itself - so here, again, we need to put the puzzle pieces together ourselves.

Hepatitis B virus (HBV) vaccination increases the risk of developing **multiple sclerosis** (MS), according to the results of a nested, case-control study published in the Sept. 14 issue of *Neurology*.

"Our analyses include 163 cases of MS and 1,604 controls," lead author Miguel A. Hernán, MD, DrPH, from the Harvard School of Public Health in Boston, Massachusetts, says in a news release. "We estimated that **immunization against hepatitis B was associated with a threefold increase in the incidence of** MS within the three years following vaccination."

Laurie Barclay, MD http://www.medscape.com/viewarticle/489057

Why would one person get MS after a hepatitis B shot and someone else not? As you can well imagine (or if you've been reading this book from the beginning), it all has to do with how much damage has already been done and where. But it may also be due to *toxic load upon the immune system*. Dr. Hal Huggins believes there is a "21 day cycle" for the immune system. If the immune system is not challenged again within 21 days of being attacked, it may be able to recover and handle the second attack. I find that very, very intriguing, since my *first* hepatitis immunization, a hepatitis A shot, was three weeks prior to the hepatitis B shot!

Revisit the chart in Chapter 3 showing how amalgams can contribute 3.8 mcg or more of mercury daily to your pollutant load. How about being injected with 12.5 mcg in a single day? It is perhaps the one single source putting hundreds, even thousands of people every year right over the top. My multiple sclerosis symptoms began within hours after a hepatitis B shot, with numbness, tingling, and twitching. Within weeks I experienced devastating depression, inability to sleep, and then muscles that felt like they were turning to rock or wood followed. I would wake up in the middle of the night to visit the bathroom, and my legs felt like they wouldn't move. It has been frightening to say the least.

We Were Told The Mercury Would Be Taken Completely Out Of Vaccines

I've seen charts generated in 2008 where pharmaceutical companies show they are taking measures to take the mercury out of vaccines. I mentioned in an earlier chapter a recent phone call to a pharmaceutical company wherein the employee admitted that many flu vaccines still contain mercury – *even when there is no thimerosal!* So if you decide to submit to a vaccination (although we also know that there is now proof that flu vaccines don't even work) make sure you at least see the ingredients on the vial. I obviously got a vial that had the mercury still in it, in 2004. The chart I saw was updated in 2008.

Mercury has been taken out of many vaccines according to the chart, but is still in some vaccines. So the onus is on you to ask to *see the label* on the bottle – don't take their word for it. Simply make sure, if you choose to vaccinate at all, that there are *no* toxins added to the bottle, no thimerosal (mercury), aluminum, formaldehyde or anything else. Know that preservatives can also be added to water that is used to "reconstitute" a dry vaccine. So be thorough in your questioning and request to see the bottle and box.

> **Thimerosal**, a derivative of mercury, is used as a preservative in hepatitis B vaccines. We measured total mercury levels before and after the administration of this vaccine in 15 preterm and 5 term infants. Comparison of pre- and **post-vaccination mercury levels showed a significant increase in both preterm and term infants after vaccination.** Additionally, post-vaccination mercury levels were significantly higher in preterm infants as compared with term infants. Because mercury is known to be a potential **neurotoxin** to infants, further study of its pharmacodynamics is warranted. [Stajich GV et al Iatrogenic exposure to mercury after hepatitis B vaccination in preterm infants. *J Pediatr* 2000 May;136(5):571-3.]

A Film From The University of Calgary in Canada: How Mercury Causes Brain Neuron Degeneration

I mentioned in Chapter 7 on *Psoriasis*, a film done by the University of Calgary called *How Mercury Causes Brain Neuron Degeneration.* This film is freely available on the internet, and is required viewing for you [go to: http://commons.ucalgary.ca/mercury/ or you can search by the title]. The film explains how even low levels of mercury (such as those that vaporize off your amalgam fillings daily) completely destroy your neurons, and thus lead to neurodegenerative disorders. If there is any time in this entire book when you *need* to understand something a bit more "technical", it is with the next section, but I've put the definition to various terms afterwards to help you.

Brain Neurons Destroyed By Mercury

Brain neurons have central cell bodies and *processes* (which basically means "arms and legs"). At the end of each neurite are growth cones where structural proteins are assembled to form the cell membrane. Two principal proteins involved are **actin** (responsible for the pulsating motion in neurons) and **tubulin**. Tubulin molecules link together to form the neurite membrane. Tubulin link together end to end to form micro tubules which surround **neurofibrils**. Growth cones in all animal species have identical structural and behavioral characteristics, using proteins of virtually identical composition. A study done by the University of Calgary (Canada) shows under the microscope, the **neurite** of a live neuron attacked by a very low concentration of mercury and destroying the **neurite membrane**, leaving behind **denuded** neurofibrils (denuded means stripped of its cover, i.e., *destroyed.*)

On the next page is a series of three photos I believe are perhaps more important than any words that could be written about mercury's neurological effects. The first photo is the healthy neuron. The second shows a tiny trace of mercury heading towards the neuron. The third photo is after the mercury has "hit" the neuron and the complete destruction that it caused. That destruction is truly only the beginning of ongoing destruction that leads to what we know as Alzheimer's, Parkinson's, multiple sclerosis, depression, ADHD, autism, Lou Gehrig's disease and so much more.

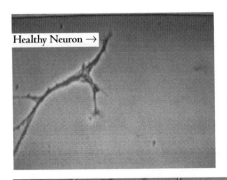

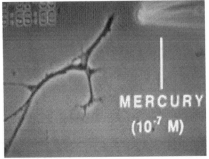

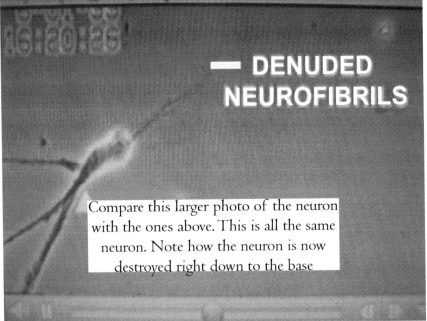

Compare this larger photo of the neuron with the ones above. This is all the same neuron. Note how the neuron is now destroyed right down to the base

Photos used by permission of Dr. Naweed I. Syed (FRCP Edin), Professor and Head Cell Biology and Anatomy, Research Director Hotchkiss Brain Institute, Faculty of Medicine, University of Calgary.

Of immense importance is that the researchers found that other toxic metals, aluminum, lead, cadmium and manganese *did not cause this effect*. This finding *should* end any and all arguments such as from your doctor or others who dismiss mercury above all other toxins as causing neurodegenerative diseases.

How Does Mercury Destroy Neurons?

The researchers explain that tubulin proteins are destroyed by mercury because mercury infiltrates the tubulin cells, attaching itself to the binding site reserved for guanosine triphosphate (GTP) on the beta subset of the tubulin molecule (which is for energy, allowing tubulin molecules to link together). Without the GTP, the mercury ions bound to these sites prevent tubulin proteins from linking together. Consequently, the tubulin then disassembles leaving the neurite stripped of its supporting structure. Ultimately the structure collapses.

This type of collapse, depending upon <u>*where*</u> it occurs in the brain or along the central nervous system is what causes the ultimate damage to brain (e.g., white matter lesions, or damage to dopamine-producing cells, or the collection of protein particles where they don't belong) i.e., all the outcomes observed in the various diseases mentioned above. In fact, the researchers talk about how research shows that animals who inhale mercury vapor go on to get lesions in the brain the same as in Alzheimer's.

Neuron the basic nerve cell of the nervous system.

Nerve any bundle of nerve fibers running to various organs and tissues of the body.

Neurite process extended by a nerve cell that can give rise to an axon or a dendrite.

Axon long, slender projection of a nerve cell or neuron that conducts electrical impulses away from the neuron's cell body.

Dendrite tree-like extension of the neuron cell body. Along with the cell body, it receives information from other neurons.

Growth cones dynamic, actin-supported extensions of a developing axon seeking its synaptic target.

Actin a contractile protein found in muscle cells.

Tubulin a globular protein that is the basic structural constituent of microtubules.

Microtubules hollow cylinders made of the protein tubulin that form, among other things, the spindle fibers.

Binding site the place on a molecule where a recognizer (protein or macromolecular complex) binds.

Denuded stripped of its cover.

Neurofibrils the cytoskeletal elements of the neuron.

Guanosine triphosphate among other things, it is used as a source of energy for protein synthesis.

Neurons connect because glutamate is released and "excites" neurons into synapsing [connecting] (see Chapter 8 *Migraines*). But when mercury damages neuron cells, the glutamatergic system (again, the amino acid transporter cells that "recycle" glutamate) as well as the immune and neurological systems go awry. With a damaged glutamate transport system, there is too much glutamate; with too much glutamate there is too much "neuro-excitement" (neurons firing wildly, even dying); with too much neuro-excitement there is a release of compounds, including nitric oxide, trying to fix the problem, and with too much nitric oxide there is widespread inflammation, pain and eventually cell death.

In addition, when protective barriers around neurons are damaged, any of a host of parasites, like herpes zoster, can, and do invade. While herpes is not the initial *cause* of MS, the virus takes its opportunity to attack and cause much misery and damage in people who have been damaged by mercury.

That Hep B Shot

I was embarking upon an Esthetician career in my early 50's, and hepatitis shots were recommended. I innocently went to get hepatitis shots, because I, like everyone else, figured it was just a dead virus that would make me "immune" to hepatitis. I was *dead* wrong. The hepatitis A shot went off without a hitch. The **hepatitis B shot** I had a few weeks later (2004) caused severe twitching down the nerve of the same arm where the shot was given and then *all hell broke loose.* When I learned there was mercury in the hepatitis B shots (none in the hepatitis A for some reason), I tried to "chelate" out the mercury (IV EDTA), but because of my kidneys' inability to excrete the mercury quick enough, the mercury was merely stirred up and redistributed. *Even worse damage occurred.* There was even worse muscle pain, unbearable cramping, weakness, depression, symptoms also of fibromyalgia, lupus (red rash on face, couldn't breathe)...*all because of mer-*

cury! It was and is devastating. More pain, more Excedrin, more kidney damage.

People who are vaccinated against **hepatitis B** are at an increased risk of developing **multiple sclerosis (MS)**, according to a study of UK patients. (My notes: This study didn't have a clue why the connection – never mentioning the high level of mercury in the vaccine) [BBC News September 14, 2004]

In August, 2006, I found myself in a lot of pain from muscles that felt as if they'd turn to wood, severe cramping, and waves of depression, this is when I went for that Tesla (the "latest") MRI and the findings were:

PATIENT NAME: TANCREDI, BARBARA

PHYSICIAN: DAVID A. STEENBLOCK, M.D.   ACCESSION #: 125075/237280

EXAM: MRI BRAIN

There are two lesions identified superiorly in the subcortical white matter of the left femoral lobe. The second lesion is in the subcortical white matter of the right front lobe

Several areas of increased signal intensity are demonstrated on long TR sequencing within the frontal lobes. There are two lesions identified superiorly in the subcortical white matter of the left femoral lobe. The second lesion is in the subcortical white matter of the right front lobe. Findings are non-specific and may be within normal limits given the patient's age. Diffusion-weighted sequencing is negative. There is no evidence of intracranial hemorrhage, mass or infarction. There are expected flow voids within the carotid and basilar arteries. The infratentorial structures are negative. There are no abnormal extra axial fluid collections. Visualized orbits and paranasal sinuses appear negative.

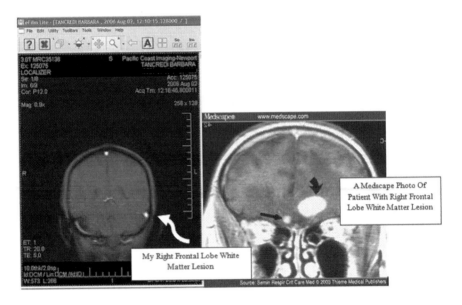

A Medscape Photo Of Patient With Right Frontal Lobe White Matter Lesion

My Right Frontal Lobe White Matter Lesion

> Multiple sclerosis is a common cause of chronic neurological disability in young adults. MRI readily identifies multifocal white matter lesions representing areas of demyelination, and is thereby useful in supporting the diagnosis of multiple sclerosis even after a single clinical episode (McDonald *et al.*, 2001).

In my own report, perhaps somewhat visible above the MRI photos, the doctor says "the findings are non-specific and may be within normal limits given the patient's age". To that I say:

1. White matter lesions are not normal as the good doctor seems to be suggesting (as if you get older it is "normal" to become pathologically damaged – it may be *common* but not "normal"). God gave you white matter – not white matter lesions.

2. When a patient comes in and plunks down hundreds or thousands of their own dollars to go through a series of MRIs (not fun) because they are suffering from waves of horrific depression, and extraordinarily painful cramping in arms, hand and feet – you don't downplay their intuition that something is wrong. The sad fact is, that if the doctor doesn't see a train wreck in your brain, he has the right to sim-

ply send the patient home without any diagnosis, much less help. Millions of people go home to suffer until what they have is as obvious as an apple-size wart on their face. This happens *more often than not.* The truth is, people are spending billions on testing and more testing in their attempt to put their finger on what is wrong with them (hoping, of course to get help!). Not only are many not getting a diagnosis, they are then not getting any medical help except "bandaids" (drugs to cover up symptoms). This is all because doctors are basically helpless – the damage has already been done. Sadly, treatment ranges from merely putting a bandaid on a gushing wound to poisoning the patient even more.

3. Unfortunately, an MRI cannot detect subtle histopathologi-cal changes that are often described as normal-appearing white matter in multiple sclerosis. This means that a patient can have all the frightening and painful symptoms – indeed, have MS, but *not* have white matter lesions – at least white matter lesions that are *visible* at the time. So to have the symptoms *and* have white matter lesions definitely points to a diagnosis of MS.

Normal-appearing **white matter** (NAWM) in established multiple sclerosis has been shown to be abnormal using a variety of magnetic resonance (MR) techniques, including proton MR spectroscopy.... [Brain, Vol. 127, No. 6, 1361-1369, 2004]

Can You Believe That Some People Still Say Mercury Isn't Toxic?

You will still hear by some people that mercury is harmless (and I guarantee you these people either have everything to gain by you not knowing the truth, *or* they are ignorant, *or* they are simply people with nothing better to do than opinionate about that which they know nothing). The truth is told in a **2006 study published in the** *Critical Review of Toxicology* where researchers rightfully state:

1. Individuals with amalgam fillings have 2-12 times more mercury in their body tissues compared to individuals without amalgams.
2. There is not necessarily a correlation between mercury levels in the blood, urine, or hair and in the body tissues, and none of the parameters correlate with severity of symptoms (My note: This means, your doctor cannot tell you whether you have mercury toxicity nor the symptoms thereof by his/her "tests" because mercury does not "hang around" in your blood, urine or hair, but will do massive damage and then "hide" deep in your bones and cells, or be escorted out of the body via detox channels.)
3. The half-life of mercury deposits in brain and bone tissues could last from several years to decades, and thus **mercury accumulates** over time of exposure.
4. Mercury, in particular mercury vapor (my note: such as that coming off of your amalgam fillings), is known to be the most toxic nonradioactive element and is toxic even in very low doses, and
5. Some studies which conclude that amalgam fillings are safe for human beings have important methodological flaws. Therefore, they have no value for assessing the safety of amalgam.

My thanks to the researchers Clarkson and Magos! [Mutter J., Naumann J., Guethlin C. Comments on the article "the toxicology of mercury and its chemical compounds" by Clarkson and Magos (2006). *Crit Rev Toxicol* 2007;37(6):537-49; discussion 551-2.] These people are obviously *truth seekers*, and know we have nothing to gain by everybody continuing to poison themselves with mercury!

Patients with certain autoimmune and allergic diseases, such as systemic lupus, **multiple sclerosis**, autoimmune thyroiditis or atopic eczema, often show increased lymphocyte stimulation by low doses of inorganic **mercury** in vitro. Mercury-containing amalgam may be an important risk factor for patients with autoimmune diseases. [Prochazkova J et al. *Neuro Endocinol Lett* 2004 Jun;25(3):211-8]

In the Prochazkova study above, my first reaction is that they're reporting the connection again, but have the cart before the horse (again) referring to *patients with autoimmune diseases* having a problem with mercury, when in fact, the mercury <u>causes</u> the autoimmune diseases!

Herpes Loves A Body Damaged By Mercury!

A migraine or MS sufferer can surely look back upon their life and tell stories of cold sores, sore throats, mumps, mono, shingles, etc. – *all caused by a virus, often the same virus!* As previously mentioned, after mercury damages the immune system, **herpes** is free to cause continuous damage and pain. Studies abound on the viral connection to multiple sclerosis. The problem is, doctors are still looking at "all the things going on" (see Chapter 5 *All The Things Going On*) and will treat you for the inflammation, the muscle cramping, the depression, etc., and never even mention, much less address, the underlying *cause* - the mercury. So people with neurological diseases go like a lamb to the slaughter when the doctor says, "okay, now its time for your flu shot".

Why are people with MS more susceptible to viral invasion and damage? It's because the protective coating around neurites is damaged, so viruses have opportunity to invade. Then with neurons and their support system damaged, nerve cells cannot travel along as they are suppose to, i.e., they have difficulty travelling from the brain to wherever their message is intended. Mixed or missing messaging is why all neurological diseases involve such symptoms as palsies (shaking), tingling, numbness, cramping, depression and so much more. All of these have to do with neurons not traveling down the "straight and narrow" pathway to an intended part of the body.

So why do viruses invade weak and damaged neurons? Viruses are known to live along nerve ganglia (a mass of nerve cells serving as a center from which nerve impulses are transmitted). The entire purpose of a virus is to replicate. If the immune and neurological system is strong, they can be kept "dormant". Once there is a weakness, they take their cue. At this point they enter cells, replicate, and in the process, injure or kill the cell. But because they are doing their dirty work along nerve ganglia, their activity is not only damaging, but also quite painful to the host - just ask anyone who has had shingles or cold sores. While shingles and cold sores are two obvious viral "outbreaks" there are *many* other painful conditions that are also viral in nature, such as chronic hip pain, trigeminal neuralgia and vertigo all of which leave most doctors baffled. (See Chapter 10 *And More*)

As I've mentioned, it is my firm conviction and experience that *every* disease starts with a pollutant and then involves an opportunistic parasite. I believe that until this becomes the *first* place doctors look, we will continue to have mismanaged, suffering people, being given one drug after another, and never really finding true healing. Even though I had cold sores often as a child, never once has a doctor connected any of my adult symptoms with a virus – even though he/she knows very well that viruses live in the host forever. For example, after the hepatitis B shot in 2004 I suddenly had a vicious bout of vertigo (severe dizziness and nausea). It kept me in bed for about three weeks! I didn't know about the mercury yet, but because I had a concurrent outbreak of genital herpes sores, I *knew* the vertigo was caused by herpes virus. In fact, I can now trace about a dozen other horrific painful attacks and nausea with herpes outbreaks that doctors never think to associate with the virus, just like the trigeminal neuralgia attack I suffered.

Herpes zoster oticus, which is caused by the spread of the **varicella-zoster virus** (shingles virus) to **facial nerves**, is characterized by intense ear pain, a rash around the ear, mouth, face, neck, and scalp, and paralysis of facial nerves. Other symptoms of herpes zoster oticus may include: hearing loss, **vertigo** (abnormal sensation of movement), tinnitus (abnormal sounds), taste loss in the tongue, dry mouth and eyes. [http://shingles.emedtv.com/herpes-zoster-oticus/herpes-zoster-oticus.html]

The fact that herpes virus is prevalent in *any* neurological disease (migraines and multiple sclerosis included) should not shock anyone. While the virus did not *cause* the disease (mercury did) it becomes of utmost importance to do everything possible to build up what is left of the body's defenses, and wage an ongoing battle to keep all viruses dormant.

1) The research findings support the presence of an increased antibody titre to **herpes virus** in the blood of **patients with MS** [*Lik Sprava.* 2004 Jan-Feb;(1):3-8]

2) It is concluded that there **is increased likelihood of HSV-2 exposure in patients with MS** [*Acta Neurol Scand.* 2006 Dec;114(6):363-7.]

3) **Varicella zoster virus (VZV), DNA was detected more frequently (P < 0.05) in the MS group (31.6%),** particularly among the relapsing-remitting MS patients (43.5%), compared with patients with other neurological diseases (10.7%). [*J Med Virol.* 2007 Feb;79(2):192-9.]

4) **DNA from varicella zoster virus (VZV) was found in 95% of MS patients** during relapse and in 17% during remission; all controls were negative; by contrast, DNA from human herpes virus 6 (HHV6) was found in 24% of MS patients during relapse and in 2% during remission; DNA from herpes simplex viruses was not found in any subject; and DNA from EBV was found in a similar percentage of subjects from all groups [*J Neurol.* 2007 Apr;254(4):493-500.]

5) We demonstrate the ability of herpes simplex virus 1 (HSV-1), human herpes virus 6 (HHV-6), and varicella zoster virus (VZV) antigens to induce higher **retrovirus reverse transcriptase** RT activity in peripheral lymphocytes from MS patients vs. controls during the first 6 days post-antigen stimulation. On subsequent days, **only VZV can sustain the increase in the RT expression in cells from MS patients.** [*J Neuroimmunol.* 2007 Jul;187(1-2):147-55.]

6) MS was relapsing-remitting at diagnosis in 136 (99%) children. The first MS attack resembled **acute disseminated encephalomyelitis** [*Lancet Neurol.* 2007 Sep;6(9):773-81.] *then, even though this study was focusing on Epstein-Barr virus, another study says:*

7) Acute Disseminated Encephalomyelitis Following *Plasmodium Falciparum* Malaria Caused By Varicella Zoster Virus Reactivation [*Am J Trop Med Hyg.*, 72(4), 2005, pp. 478-480]

Scientists historically spend decades studying various things going on in a disease in order to prove it to be the "cause". When they can't prove that one thing going on to be the cause they often abandon the theory and move onto the next thing going on. Again, the truth is that mercury damaged the immune system of the MS sufferer, and *any* virus will become opportunistic and begin a feeding frenzy on the body. Remember, the virus is merely being found at "the scene of the crime". I've had viral problems since I was a small child with horrific outbreaks of cold sores, for example, that would spread across my entire cheek. Only after a hepatitis B shot as a 51 year old did I get MS.

Herpes itself doesn't cause MS. The domino effect of "things going on" is started by mercury, and that is the most important factor here worth repeating until we're confused no longer. Indeed, until this fact is fully understood and acknowledged, we will not stop the statistical fact that every other person is being badly damaged by mercury.

I also repeat that this is not to discount viruses. Viruses are the bain of human existence and must be dealt with on a daily basis. Viral activity results in pustular lesions, extreme pain (I repeat, they live along nerves!), inflammation, fever, vertigo, hearing loss, hip pain, further damage to body cells and tissues, and cancer. Many people live their entire lives with dormant viruses that may only cause an occasional cold sore – or nothing. There is no question that viruses cause damage to your body. MS would be an entirely different disease if herpes weren't there doing massive damage to cells.

To reiterate:
1. For many, MS can start immediately after a hepatitis B shot. In the past hepatitis B shots had the highest amount of mercury, a whopping 12.5 mcg per injection – *and* hepatitis immunization is given in a series only a few weeks apart (not giving your body any time to recover from the first toxic

onslaught). But of course, *any* vaccine with mercury in it will do damage – as can ingestion of mercury "over the top" from any source.

2. You may have had herpes (I, II, zoster) all your life, but after mercury, when at your weakest, shingles or any other exacerbation can cause much damage and much misery. Herpes definitely makes multiple sclerosis and all other diseases worse.

3. Brains and bodies damaged by mercury are further damaged by free glutamates. Migraines and MS are caused by mercury's damage to DNA, mitochondria, the immune system and the glutamatergic system.

Most People Have Herpes!

Scientists tell us that *most* Americans have herpes. I was listening to Dr. Laura in the summer of 2008 and a young woman called in sobbing that she'd just been diagnosed with herpes simplex II (genital herpes). She sobbed as if her life was over. All I know is that Dr. Laura allowed this girl to sob without *ever* comforting her telling her that approximately 40,000 people are infected with just HSV-I (herpes simplex virus I - the kind that causes "cold sores") *every day*. It has also been published that 80% of all people have herpes and in other publications I've read that 95% have herpes. The high percentage is understandable considering the fact that there are many different types of herpes from HSV-I (cold sores), HSV-2 (genital herpes), and varicella zoster (shingles) and more.

Here's the important thing Dr. Laura failed to comfort this young woman with (but this is also a failure of most healthcare professionals): If your immune system is strong, you can actually live your entire life without having herpes rear it's ugly head and cause you misery, damage and even death (e.g., from cancer). But when your immune system is badly damaged by heavy metals, especially mercury, the herpes living dormant in you can now cause massive harm and indescribable pain. The best thing this young woman could have been told is *don't ever get another flu shot or vaccination with thimerosal, don't eat fish, don't get amalgam fillings and don't smoke (cadmium).* She also should have been told to avoid high arginine foods (like chocolate and nuts) and to take lysine! That sobbing young woman acted as if she'd been given a death sentence and it's simply not true. We don't just walk around innocently minding our own business and have viruses come and bite us out of the blue. Viruses can live *dormant* in you for your entire lifetime. Viruses have likely existed since Adam and Eve ate the forbidden apple (it's all their fault).

…increased antibody titre to herpes virus in the blood of patients with MS. [Kruhliak HO et al., Multiple sclerosis and herpetic infection *Lik Sprava.* 2004 Jan-Feb;(1):3-8.]

…high frequency of **varicella zoster virus** (the one that causes shingles) DNA in the cerebrospinal fluid of patients with multiple sclerosis [*J Med Virol.* 2007 Feb;79(2):192-9]

DNA from **varicella zoster virus** was found in 95% of MS patients during relapse and in 17% during remission [*J Neurol.* 2007 Apr;254(4):493-500.]

MS in children might be associated with exposure to **Epstein Barr Virus** (EBV) [*Lancet Neurol.* 2007 Sep;6(9):773-81.]

There have been a variety of viruses found in MS patients. This fact supports my own findings that viruses are opportunistic and feed upon diseased cells instead of the other way around. Since I've had many outbreaks of various viruses for my entire lifetime, but only "got" multiple sclerosis right after a mercury injection, I am *completely* convinced – but all of the science should convince you as well. *Mercury* causes multiple sclerosis. No mercury = No multiple sclerosis.

The Glutamatergic System Is Also Damaged In MS

We discussed how mercury damages the glutamatergic system and thus causes migraines. But the glutamatergic system is also damaged in victims with MS. Indeed, glutamate elevation is found in both migraines and multiple sclerosis (and, as would follow, in many (if not all) neurological diseases). High glutamate levels lead to **central nervous system "lesions"** (damaged areas) which cause interference of normal neuron signals. You'll often hear about damage to the myelin sheath in multiple sclerosis. *Lesions* are created along this neuron signalling pathway. Think of it like a huge pile of bricks you might encounter on a walk and you can't get around that pile. Neural passage can also be impeded causing neurons to stop, go off path, pile up and tangle.

In MS, the immune system attacks the white matter of the brain and spinal cord... **glutamate levels are increased in acute MS lesions** and in normal-appearing white matter in MS patients... factors which may contribute to perturbing glutamate homeostasis include altered activity of the glutamate-producing enzyme glutaminase... and altered expression of the glutamate transporters EAAT-1 and EAAT-2 (Note: EAAT = excitotoxic amino acid transporter and is part of what makes up the *glutamatergic system* we talk about being damaged) [C. Matute et al. Increased expression and function of white matter injury by glutamate. *J Neurosci* 25, 2952–2964. 2007]

Glutamate damages the myelin sheath.

Injury to oligodendrocyte progenitors, caused in part by **glutamate** and the subsequent derailment of Ca 2+ homeostasis, contributes to the pathogenesis of **myelination disturbances** in this illness (speaking of multiple sclerosis) [Back & Rivkees, 2004].

and

In MS, the immune system attacks the **white matter** of the brain and spinal cord, leading to disability and/or paralysis. Myelin and oligodendrocytes are lost due to the release by immune cells of cytotoxic cytokines, autoantibodies and **toxic amounts of glutamate** [Matute et al. 2001; Srinivasan et al. 2005].

Stop Consuming Free Glutamates

In Chapter 11 *Nature's Medicines,* I explain what you can do to slow and God-willing, halt the progression of MS. There are lifestyle choices, dietary choices, supplements and natural therapies you need to know about. Avoiding free glutamates is absolutely essential for *anyone...*but especially for anyone with a brain and body damaged by mercury.

Glutathione Is Depleted In MS

Mercury exerts a variety of toxic effects in the body. Lipid peroxidation, **DNA damage** and **depletion of reduced glutathione by Hg(II)** suggest an oxidative stress-like mechanism for Hg(II) toxicity. [*Basic & Clinical Pharmacology & Toxicology,* Volume 93, Number 6, December 2003 , pp. 290-296(7)]

Glutathione is a powerful compound in the body made up of amino acids (building blocks of proteins). Glutathione protects your cells against the damaging effects of oxidation. It has a synergistic effect with other antioxidants to protect the body against free radicals and oxidizing agents that cause so much damage to the body through what is commonly referred to as 'oxidative stress'. Glutathione attaches itself to toxic chemicals and drugs in the liver and renders them into a state suitable for elimination from the body. These toxic materials include poisonous pesticides, hydrogen sulfide, carbon monoxide, toxic metals such as mercury, cadmium and chromium and many other substances that we come into contact with due to present day pollution of our atmosphere and foodstuffs. The reason the study mentioned in the box above says that one of mercury's toxic effects is to deplete glutathione is because it gets "used up" trying to protect you from the mercury. How to increase your body's glutathione is explained in Chapter 11 *Nature's Medicines.*

With MS There Can Be Great Difficulty Relaxing and Sleeping

One dreadful part of MS is difficulty relaxing and falling asleep. You need a healthy glutamatergic system to make gamma amino-butyric acid (GABA), in order to have restful, normal sleep. GABA is the most important inhibitory neurotransmitter in the brain. It's job is to induce relaxation and sleep. Where "exicitation" occurs in the brain, GABA is supposed to be there to provide the opposite effect, or the "calm". People with multiple sclerosis are deficient in GABA. It's not just people with MS that have difficulty falling asleep, so do people with most neurological diseases. Television commercials of one new sleep aid after another tell the sad tale. We have a nation of people getting neurological diseases and we have a nation of people having trouble going to sleep – and all because of every level of neurological damage caused mostly by mercury, pesticides and glutamates, which inhibit the normal function and production of glutamates and thus GABA in the brain (and all that this affects). Unfortunately, taking GABA is not the answer because *it's made from glutamate.* It would be yet another supplement that could cause further problems in some-one with a damaged glutamatergic system. Fortunately studies show melatonin apparently takes the place of GABA in inducing sleep. See melatonin section in Chapter 11 *Nature's Medicines.*

> GABA (gamma-aminobutyric acid) is naturally made in the brain from the amino acid glutamate, helped by vitamin B6. It is the brain's chief 'inhibitory' neurotransmitter, known to help induce relaxation, analgesia, and sleep. [by John W Winkelman, MD, PhD, et al. November 13, 2008]

The Most Important Things You Can Do

Before knowing what to do I carried on in life, though handi-capped in so many ways. I no longer tried to hold down a full-time job *outside* of my home because I was never able to predict what kind of pain I would wake up to or be slapped with mid-day. I learned to work at shorter tasks even though I was having a horrific migraine or suffering from debilitating fatigue from the MS. I took so much Excedrin my kidneys hurt chronically, so I went to a nephrologist to have them monitored (I didn't have insurance, so I paid for this myself). At 52 I was told they were about 60% damaged. Then, after a kidney test at age 53 the doctor would no longer tell me the results, but behaved as if he was very concerned. He told me, "perhaps you need a different doctor". (I've heard that before – they're thinking – "this lady's bad off, she doesn't have any insurance – send her somewhere else quick!")

When I didn't yet know about mercury in amalgams nor in immunizations, I found myself looking for the same things doctors look for, i.e., what to do to ameliorate symptoms. The medical symptom/ treatment hype is so convincing even I fell temporarily prey. I went to doctors dozens of times looking for help. So now here I am in my 50's and insurance companies won't give me insurance. They say I "go to doctors too much", and am considered a "major risk". *But it's* their *fault.* I can't even express the lifetime of suffering I've experienced. What I *can* express is that:

Much suffering has been contributed to or even caused by the poor decisions of many leaders in the very medical and government agencies who are supposed to be helping, **not hurting us.**

We must no longer merely assume that something we're told to do is safe (for example when your doctor says, "So, Mrs. So-and-so, are you ready for that flu shot?"). Neither can we simply trust someone just because they have a medical degree or stand behind a pharmaceutical counter. In addition it is your responsibility to eat right, take the right supplements and maintain other healing practices. You cannot "claim ignorance" nor cover your ears, loudly singing "La, La, La", with a candy bar in hand, while someone is trying to advise you on the virtues of consuming organic fruit instead. Making the best of choices can keep you functioning and enjoying life. You will find there will be no one to blame but yourself when you suffer because of making bad choices. Yes, the government watchdogs as well as medical professionals *should* pay attention (we've known about the toxicity of mercury since antiquity!) but if *they* don't, *you* must! Many right choices are more thoroughly explained in Chapter 11 *Nature's Medicines.*

First – Keep educating yourself about **the dangers of mercury**, and of course never, ever allow it to be put into your body in any way: Not by injections, amalgams, eating fish, breaking a flourescent or "long-life bulb", in makeup or medicines, etc. Learn all the sources and do everything in your power to stay away from mercury. Of course you want to stay away from *all* toxic metals like aluminum, lead and arsenic as well.

Second – Adopt a pure, whole, fresh, (preferably organic) plant foods diet as the bulk of your diet. Also make sure that any other foods you eat contain absolutely **no glutamates** and **no pesticides**. On this diet you will be supplying your body with copious amounts of phytochemicals which, as you now know, are *vital* to healing and maintaining health. Also in these raw fruits and vegetables are over 6,000 compounds, each of which has near miraculous functions within the body – not the least of which would be to protect you from mercury and other toxins and even stimulate your own stem cells to heal you.

Third – Take **CaAEP** daily on a schedule. A suggestion would be 2 capsules every 4 hours. You can increase the dose as needed. At the same time, take the **anti-inflammatory herbs and supplements** recommended in Chapter 11 *Nature's Medicines.*

Fourth – Take the anti-fungal, viral, bacterial supplements suggested in Chapter 11 *Nature's Medicines.* To help keep herpes at bay, *never* eat nuts, seeds, chocolate or glutenous grains (your starches are potatoes, yams, corn and rice).

Fifth – **Walk and Sun** every single day that you can, allowing your bare skin to soak up the sun. If you can work up a sweat, all the better.

Chapter 10
AND MORE

Hip Pain

How many people do you know who suffer from hip pain? I have suffered since my late 20's with severe hip pain. I used to say that when I bent over it was like someone stabbing me with a hot poker in the hip. Through the years I went to doctor after doctor. None had any idea what was wrong, because I didn't have clicking, grinding, popping or difficulty walking (indications of a hip joint needing a replacement). All I had was horrible pain that would keep me up nights. I had to take pain medication. One doctor I went to, after I pointed out where the pain was, had the audacity to proclaim "there's nothing there!" I was pointing to my buttock, down into the hip joint. I didn't know enough at the time to say anything, but if that happened to me today, I'd say…"what about my hip joint, or the sciatic nerve that's as thick as your finger running down through that hip joint???"

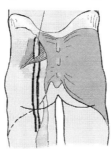

Drawing of the hip and the placement of the sciatic nerve running down through the hip joint. Dark gray is depiction of muscle that, on the left side, has been "stripped away" to reveal the sciatic nerve.

It wasn't until my early 50's that I finally figured it out. It was after having suffered for the first time with an *outbreak* of **herpes zoster, shingles**, that had broken out on the back of my thigh. Understand that I've had herpes zoster all my life, ever since having chicken pox while elementary school age. Viruses live in you for your entire life. But this was the first time since the chicken pox that the symptoms were *visible*. There were itching, aching and burning sores all over the back of my thigh. I suffered a concomitant spell of severe hip pain. Ah-ha! Herpes resides dormant *in your nerves*, rising in times of low-ered immunity and stress to rear its ugly and painful head. So why is the pain so severe in the hip? It's because herpes is residing in the sciatic nerve, I repeat, a nerve as thick as your finger. And the nerve runs right down through your hip. Big nerve = big pain. That ex-plains having this hip pain since my 20's and no-one having a clue as to how, why, or what.

Normally I'd suffer the hip pain for weeks, even months. This time, instead of fighting just the pain, which I'd done for 30+ years, now I fought the virus, and the hip pain went away in days. Now I found I could keep the pain away for months at a time. In fact, I work hard at keeping all viruses dormant. Because of mercury damage, her-pes attacks (and I've shown symptoms and have had blood tests show-ing I have at least herpes I, 2, and zoster) are more frequent.

What I use to keep herpes under control is outlined in Chapter I I *Nature's Medicines.* At one point I tried a prescription, Acyclovir, but learned that it is very hard on the kidneys, and the assault on my kidneys was immediate. I became very ill after just one pill. I was reminded that dangerous drugs are not the answer. There are power-ful natural supplements and therapies that ultimately work far safer. For example, I purchased a T.E.N.S Unit (stands for Transcutaneous Electrical Nerve Stimulation). T.E.N.S. devices deliver mild electrical pulses through the skin to stimulate the cutaneous (surface) and affer-ent (deep) nerves to help control pain. Unlike the danger of too many pain medications, T.E.N.S. does not have any known side effects. But they can be expensive. I found one at www.medicalproductsonline.org for under $100.00 (normally $500.00).

Vertigo

I awoke one morning, within that first year of having the symptoms of MS, unable to get out of bed. The room was spinning in large circles, and I was horrifically nauseous. This went on for about three weeks! I knew it was **vertigo**, but I had no idea what caused it, until towards the end when I had a herpes II outbreak and hip pain. Herpes! My husband has had many bouts of vertigo which sent him to bed for days, to suffer horrible nausea and vomiting, along with a migraine-like headache.

Realizing there are many potential "manifestations" of herpes, I became even stricter about avoiding high arginine foods. This tactic can keep herpes dormant, and nitric oxide levels down. Then, in 2008 I celebrated my 55th birthday with my daughter, and she made "organic" hamburgers. I had a whole wheat bun. Normally, I never eat grains – too high in arginine. The next day I broke out with a herpes II outbreak. Not long after this was Thanksgiving. We celebrated, as usual, at another daughter's home. There are so many choices, I never have trouble filling a plate. I had fresh roasted turkey (no seasonings are put on it), yams I brought and had cooked in olive oil with onions and "orange zest", a fresh cranberry relish made of ground cranberries and oranges and a little sugar. I never eat the "stuffing" – full of seasonings and grains, even nuts. But I also never eat the mashed potatoes because the person who makes them uses many seasonings and margarine (glutamates). Likewise, I don't have the gravy she seasons. But I had a salad with organic olive oil and rice vinegar only. It was made especially for us with organic baby greens and lots of other goodies....but they'd also put in pine nuts. I didn't bother to take them out – it was Thanksgiving!

The next morning I awoke to a spinning room again, and horrific nausea. I crawled to the bathroom and took four 500 mg. vege-cap pills of L-Lysine (an arginine opposer), 500 mg. of vitamin C, and used "Insure Herbal" tincture (echinacea-goldenseal mixture) in water to take the pills. I crawled back to bed, back to sleep, and awoke several hours later. The vertigo and nausea were about 90% gone. I took the same pills and herbal formula, this time with four pro-biotic (acidophilus) capsules. I ate a banana (tough to do when you're even a little nauseous) and took four ginger capsules (vegetarian capsules because gelatin ones contain free glutamates). Within an hour I was able to function normally.

My research confirmed what I suspected: My vertigo was from a herpes outbreak in the ear area. It took another few weeks of intense anti-viral use to get over this bout completely, but this time I wasn't bed-ridden nor felt so badly I couldn't function. What a contrast to years ago when I didn't have a clue what the vertigo was caused by, and suffered horrifically for so many days. (See Chapter 11 *Nature's Medicines* for more explanation as to how and why these supplements work.)

While I don't claim to have suffered or to currently suffer "Ramsay Hunt Syndrome" it proves the reality that herpes infection in the ear area causes vertigo. Since all herpes viruses live along nerves, I believe *any* herpes virus, whether I, II, zoster, etc. can take up residence anywhere in the body causing the myriad of symptoms to which we assign disease names. In fact, it often occurs to me that we're confusing matters by calling this virus *herpes zoster oticus* as if it's a different virus than herpes zoster. It is not. It's the same virus that causes shingles. The importance of this is that if people would realize that once they have a virus they have it for their entire life, they will better understand that the virus can spread throughout the body causing a variety of diseases all in the same person.

In one person, herpes zoster can contribute to trigeminal neuralgia, tinnitus, vertigo, hearing loss, eye infections, shingles, hip pain *and more.* Why is this so very important? Because you need to fight the *virus* NOT run to the doctor for each of these symptoms and take a drug or perform some surgical procedure for each one. This is where we do ourselves great harm. Not only are we *not* addressing the underlying virus, but we're adding great insult to the injury already going on. Of course I have to say it again — if there'd been no damage by mercury, the virus wouldn't have such an opportunity to wreck such havoc.

> Herpes zoster oticus (also known as Ramsay Hunt Syndrome or Ramsay Hunt Syndrome type II) is an infection caused by the varicella-zoster virus. *Herpes zoster oticus is infection of the 8th cranial nerve ganglia and the geniculate ganglion of the facial nerve by the herpes zoster virus.* Symptoms of herpes zoster oticus include hearing loss, **vertigo**, and tinnitus. [http://shingles.emedtv.com/herpes-zoster-oticus/herpes-zoster-oticus.html]

Trigeminal Neuralgia

I had a horrific bout of **trigeminal neuralgia** as I explained in Chapter 6 *Dental Work*. It is explained in that chapter because people who suffer from it feel like every tooth in their jaw needs a root canal. It's a common misconception, and people do end up with unecessary, painful, expensive root canals (which, especially with immune problems, end up rotting and contribute further to neurological diseases — also explained in this book) or they end up having teeth pulled in an attempt to end the horrific pain!

Trigeminal neuralgia was by far the worst pain I have ever suffered in my life. For someone who has suffered 10+ chronic migraines, MS, ulcers and more, *that's saying a lot.* It was as if a gun was being fired point blank at my jaw every 30 seconds. It started suddenly. I awoke to "shot gun" pain in my jaw. It radiated up into my ear, into the right side of my head. I felt as if I needed a root canal in every tooth on that side of my head — upper and lower jaw! I ran to my car and drove, sobbing, to my "holistic" dentist — I could barely see the road because of the horrendous pain. He took me in and through sobs I asked him, "what is this???" He looked perplexed. He clearly didn't know. He tapped my teeth as I begged him to anesthetize my entire jaw so I could think straight…so I could get some relief. I felt like I would die from the stress of the pain! I'd taken an Excedrin that works about 50% of the time for my migraines at the time, but it did absolutely nothing for this pain.

It wasn't long before the dentist was perturbed with me. He was irritated and said, "well, what do you want *me* to do? Do you want me to start a root canal?" I told him I didn't know which tooth would need it...they all felt as if they did. Still unhappy (I was clearly interrupting his normal schedule) he said, "well which tooth hurts the *most?*" I pointed to number 5. He immediately began a root canal. I walked out of that office in as much pain as when I went in...even after that root canal!

It's a few years later. I've now lost tooth number 5, and am quickly losing number 6 (my canine!) and number 4 as well – all because of that unnecessary root canal. I'm in a "dental crises" in good part because that dentist didn't have a *clue* what the symptoms of trigeminal neuralgia are and did a root canal on me – a root canal I've since had to pull out. Then, in order to place a bridge, a different dentist prepped the tooth on either side of number 5. As I write this I'm sitting with a temporary bridge over those three spots because they're not doing well. They all ache. All this because a medical professional didn't know what trigeminal neuralgia is.

The "rabbit" (See Chapter 5 *All The Things Going On*) in trigeminal neuralgia is damage to neurons, the glutamatergic system, and the immune system by **mercury**. With the immune system damaged, viruses proliferate along nerve ganglia - the most painful place they could possibly exist. When even the little defense you have left is "down", these viruses replicate out of control along the nerves, causing pain like none other. If you're doing nothing to fight viruses naturally, and build up what immune system you have left, you can have a very painful life, indeed.

This all began to happen after I started having flu shots and that hepatitis B shot. How about you, did you have your flu shot this year? Last year? I foolishly did, for two years in a row. *But never again!* Mercury does rapid and irreversible damage, and then hides where normal tests do not detect it.

Once neurons and the immune system are damaged, opportune viruses invade and live dormant along your nerves for your entire life. It can be zoster or I or II....I don't think anyone knows for sure, and frankly it doesn't matter! When the virus activates the pain is often excrutiating. This is because nerves are so sensitive (nerves are how you feel even a feather as it touches your skin!)

The trigeminal nerve is made up of three branches (hence "tri") and run down along your teeth as well as up into your head. So the pain feels as though all of your teeth are in need of root canals, your ear aches, and your head aches right to the core of your brain. It's excrutiating, and no normal analgesics offer any relief. People go to their perplexed doctors and get dangerous drugs and powerful pain killers like morphine. Some resort to root canals or having teeth pulled, while all along it's a virus. None of what the doctors prescribe or do eradicates the virus.

I had an "outbreak" of trigeminal neuralgia *once.* Once is enough. I pray daily, Lord, please don't *ever* let me drop my guard and let that happen again. I had an unnecessary root canal that is giving me hell now, not to mention literally thousands upon thousands of dollars in attempts to repair.

Tonsillitis

From the age of 11 on, I have had recurring tonsillitis. I was sick more often than not in both middle school and high school. I had normal attendance in elementary school prior to the mercury poisoning. In fact, if you know someone who seems to always have some kind of infection, look for the mercury, and damage to their immune system. Never in my 55 years did I think of my tonsillitis being connected to the herpes and the mercury damage. But of course it was.

Just to share a funny story, I recall going to a school doctor in college and seeing him write "necrotic" on the paper. Seeing it upside-down I thought he wrote neurotic! For weeks until I went back and bravely insisted they let me see my chart, I thought the doctor saw me as neurotic! (See text box next page)

> We present a case report of a 22-year-old woman with bilateral cervical adenopathy, **acute tonsillitis**, and suspected peritonsillar abscess. Histologic examination of the excised tonsils demonstrated discrete **necrotic areas** that contained cells with intranuclear viral inclusions. The diagnosis of **herpetic tonsillitis** was confirmed by demonstrating herpes simplex virus (HSV)-infected cells on paraffin section immunostains and by positive HSV cultures of the tonsillar tissue. [Mayo Clin Proc 1994 Mar;69(3):269-71]

Tonsillitis is *not* just a normal part of growing up. I raised three kids and in those 20 glorious years my children did not have the usual childhood diseases and suffering. My eldest daughter had a single bout of sore throat (was sick for a few weeks) my son has had sore throats off and on during his 23 years, and my youngest had no illnesses to speak of as a young child and only bladder infections occasionally as an adult. I hear of child after child in other families where routine doctor visits and careful adherence to immunizations takes place (mercury!) who have diabetes, asthma, childhood cancers etc.

My children were *not* immunized. When all the other kids were getting measles, mumps, etc., they got "a spot" and simply stayed home from school for a few days playing happily until the "outbreak" was over. That spot told me they had encountered the virus or bacteria and it "immunized" them the way God intended – by a healthy immune system encountering the bug, building up antibodies and making them even stronger. But this only works if the immune system hasn't first been damaged by mercury!

Children, often from the better families who have enough money to run to the doctor or emergency room for "all the recommended" immunizations and doctor care, are all too often rushed as infants and small children to the emergency room with horrific fevers, stopped up breathing and near-death experiences. My children never even came close to being rushed to the emergency room with any of those things. I was from a less affluent family and wasn't taken to the doctor but maybe once or twice in my childhood. It was only *after* the age of eleven, and after my mouthful of amalgams that I suffered appreciable illness as a young child, like frequent strep throat and eye sties. Then came the psoriasis, of course.

Without question, my tonsillitis was *caused* by a damaged immune system, damaged by mercury. The opportune parasite was herpes. When I got tonsillitis I would have those "necrotic" areas on my tonsils, and concurrent "cold sores".

Tinnitus – *Ringing In The Ears*

Ever experienced a sudden loud noise and your ears "rang" afterwards? Even hurt?! Firecrackers, gunshots, a smoke detector going off near your head – any of these and more can lead to temporary ear pain and ringing. The fact is, injury to the neurological workings of the ear, whether temporary or long-term is what causes ringing. If you go to the doctor you'll be told nobody knows what causes chronic ringing, yet science shows us it's neurological damage. So the question is really, is it temporary or permanent? And what is wrecking havoc with the neurological workings of the ear(s)?

What wrecks havoc and causes *all* diseases are pollutants and parasites. If you suffer chronic ringing in the ears you'll want to determine what's causing that ringing so it won't lead to deafness. So its your job to discern which pollutant and/or which parasite is likely causing your problem. Mercury is the #1 known damager of neurons. Have you had recent amalgam fillings? How about a flu shot or other immunization? Have you been in a room where an "energy saving" lightbulb or flourescent lightbulb broke (mercury)? Have you been eating fish? Shark and swordfish are high in mercury and all fish contain some level of mercury!

Of course working around loud noise all day could do the damage as well. The studies below show that tinnitus (and other problems in the eye and ear area) has a herpes connection. "Sudden deafness" has been scientifically shown to be due to damage that herpes can do to the nerve.

The greatest liklihood of chronic ringing in the ears, if not caused by an *acoustic* blast of some kind (like daily loud noises at work, or a major blast right by your ears, etc.), is a herpes infection. By far the best way to prevent hearing loss is never getting any mercury, and by taking immune-enhancing, viral-fighting supplements, like "Insure Herbal" (a combination of echinacea and goldenseal), vitamin C, astragalus, L-lysine and colloidal silver.

If you suspect a viral component, and well you should, take four 500 mg. (vegetable capsules) of lysine with a glass of water on an empty stomach at least three times a day until you're better. This could take a day to a month. After your symptoms subside take the lysine and other supplements "periodically" on a regular schedule to keep the virus dormant. Also do not consume nuts, seeds, and chocolate, as these are extraordinarily high in arginine, the amino acid that fuels the growth and replication of viruses (and cancer cells). Grains are also high in arginine, try to eat non-glutenous grains most of the time, like millet and rice. Substitute potatoes, yams and corn for your starch needs.

Never use cortisone when you suspect a viral or fungal outbreak, as steroids make these infections much worse. Acyclovir is a prescription medication for viruses, but is very hard on the kidneys, and I'm not the only one that says it doesn't work any better than that outlined above.

1. ...**tinnitus**, neuritis, hearing impairment – infection with **varicella zoster virus** [*Acta Otorrinolaringol Esp.* 2006 Apr;57(4):189-92]

2. ...**tinnitus** – **Herpes Simplex** Virus IgG and IgM were positive – probably immune deficiency [*Acta Medica (Hradec Kralove). 2004;47(1):55-8.*]

3. ...viral labyrinthitis, sudden sensioneural hearing loss – **herpes family** [*Ann Otol Rhinol Laryngol.* 2003 Nov;112(11):993-1000.]

4. ...**tinnitus** – **zoster oticus** [*J Neurol Neurosurg Psychiatry.* 2001 Aug;71(2):149-54.]

5. ...**tinnitus** – an etiological role for the **herpes virus family** is assumed. [*Acta Otolaryngol.* 1998 Jul;118(4):488-95.]

6. ...**tinnitus** – **varicella-zoster virus** – infection originates in the cranial ganglia. [*Rinsho Shinkeigaku.* 1995 Jul;35(7):814-6.]

7. ...tinnitus – varicella zoster virus. [*Ann Neurol.* 1994;35 Suppl:S62-4.]
8. ...tinnitus, sudden, unexpected hearing loss – herpetic [*J Laryngol Otol.* 1990 Feb;104(2):104-8.]
9. ...tinnitus – herpes oticus [*Acta Otolaryngol Suppl.* 1984;419:163-6.]
10. ...deafness occurred in association with herpes zoster ophthalmicus. [*Arch Dermatol.* 1983 Mar;119(3):235-6.]
11. Auditory symptoms associated with herpes zoster [*Laryngoscope.* 1977 Mar;87(3):372-9.]
12. A case of herpes zoster on the trunk with affliction of the acoustic nerve. [*Sb Ved Pr Lek Fak Karlovy Univerzity Hradci Kralove.* 1969;12(2):189-91.]

Ulcers

When I was in my 30's I awoke one work-day morning, unable to get up and get ready for work. My stomach was churning, on fire, and I was in horrific pain. I was doubled over on my bed, not knowing what was causing it. As fate (actually God) would have it, I was working full-time as a nutritionist at the time, and had access to the best advice. I called Dr. Michael Murray (naturopathic doctor and professor at Bastyr University) and described the problem. He told me it was ulcers and told me to take DGL. I had never heard of it. He told me it was deglycyrrhizinated licorice. That is, they took out the glycerritinic acid from licorice because it can cause a fluctuation in blood pressure, but left the other parts. When chewed and mixed with saliva the licorice goes to work healing the mucosal lining of the entire gastrointestinal tract. I began taking DGL immediately. After chewing up just a few of the tablets the pain was gone. I've been using it ever since, every time I have the least symptom of stomach pain.

You may hear that ulcers are caused by *helicobactor pylori*. But the truth is, we find *helicobactor pylori* at the scene of the crime. It doesn't *cause* the crime. *Pollutants* are the true underlying cause of diseases. *Parasites* are opportunistic. Parasites, like *helicobactor pylori* see an opportune time to invade when your cells are damaged, and do so. Most people only look at "all the things going on" then blame the parasites for causing the disease. In the case of ulcers, *acids* cause the damage to the gastrointestinal lining. These acids can come from extreme stress (excess HCl), aspirin and other drugs like cortisone, or even a horrific diet high in chemicals like MSG and trans fats. So the "rabbit" is *acid*. *Helicobactor pylori* is merely at the scene of the crime, taking the opportunity to invade after the stomach cells have been damaged.

How do I know? Because time and time again I've had a flare up of my ulcers after using cortisone, aspirin or when under intense stress. We *all* have bacteria,viruses and fungus in us at all times. It's only when our defenses are down that they are able to invade, and they invade diseased tissue. The only exception to parasites being *more* than merely opportunistic might be with the most virulent viruses, like AIDS (which many say is a man-made virus). But even the AIDS virus is warded off by the healthiest individuals for quite some time.

Avoiding the acids and caustic substances that damage the GI lining is the first course of action. DGL is the second. I've had a flair up of my ulcers only a few times since that initial introduction to them, and every time I was able to heal them over by chewing up as many DGL as I needed. This, too, is the beauty of God's medicines, not only do they work to heal (not just put a band-aid over the problem), but you can almost always take as much as you need, whenever you need. On the other hand, a relative of mine had stomach pain and the doctor gave him Prilosec (a drug for hyper acidity). He took it happily for years so happy to not suffer any more pain, and you might say, "who could blame him?" When he was told he had cancer, it was all throughout his gut. If you have pain anywhere, you need to find out what is causing it and correct what is wrong, not cover it up with a drug, or it will develop into far worse things.

Chapter 11
NATURE'S MEDICINES

The important points in this chapter are the ways you can address both the cause *and* "all the things going on" in migraines, multiple sclerosis and more. The dietary factors, supplements and other measures are for:

1 – Eliminating all mercury, free glutamates and pesticides (and other toxins)

2 – Saturating the body with the over 6,000 known phytonutrients designed to strengthen and protect the body's cells

3 – Utilizing powerful supplements that are: Anti-inflammatory (oppose nitric oxide and other inflammatory compounds) and, anti-viral (as well as anti-fungal and anti-bacterial)

4 – Utilizing supplements for general immune-enhancement, healing and to address symptoms

The Difference Between Nature's Medicines And Man's Medicines

The difference between Nature's medicines (which I unapologetically personally refer to as "God's medicines") and man's medicines is this: Man harnesses and combines various chemicals in an attempt to stop something going on in the body. Because man is *not* all-knowing, all-seeing, nor all-understanding, man can generally only target one thing at a time. For example, man has searched and discovered after much searching that there are proteins called "Cyclooxygenase" or "Cox" for short. Read definition below:

> **Cox-2:** Cyclooxygenase-2, a protein that acts as an enzyme and specifically catalyzes (speeds) the production of certain chemical messengers called prostaglandins. Some of these messengers are responsible for **promoting inflammation.** When Cox-2 activity is blocked, inflammation is reduced. Unlike Cox-1, Cox-2 is active only at the site of inflammation, not in the stomach. [http://www.medicinenet.com/nonsteroidal_antiinflammatory_drugs/glossary.htm]

After discovering "Cox", man discovered a chemical that is a "Cox-2 inhibitor", and thus stops inflammation because it targets the Cox-2 protein. Unfortunately, Cox-1 is also targeted by these inhibitors, and Cox-1 is a protein that produces *protective* chemicals within the body. The various Cox-2 inhibitors include aspirin, acetaminophen, Vioxx, Celebrex, paracetamol, and more. Most people have heard of the problems with the stronger prescription Cox-2 inhibitors. People have been harmed and have even died.

But the problem with the daily, fairly unrestricted use of certain Cox-2 inhibitors known as "NSAIDS" (non-steroidal antiinflammatory drugs) applies to *all* drugs. The truth is, when man ingests a chemical designed to target one specific thing within the body, that chemical does not simply behave itself, go right to where man wants it to go, do the job, and do nothing else. Unfortunately, that chemical goes *all over the body* and can cause harm where it was never intended to go. This is why drugs can and do cause widespread damage.

Don't believe me? The next time you listen to a commercial about a drug, listen closely to the end of the commercial where they rattle off all the "potential, but rare" side-effects. They are frightening! "coma", "death", "hemorrhage", "lupus", "cancer", "blood clots", "stroke". As mentioned in a previous chapter, these so-called "rare" side-effects are *not rare at all.* Prove it to yourself. Now with the internet you can go into "chat rooms" with regard to almost every drug and find thousands of people crying out for help. These people have connected the drug they were prescribed and taking with new and worse diseases they are now suffering.

In particular, the risk of serious **cardiovascular thrombotic events**, e.g. **myocardial infarction**, was 1.7% in the **Vioxx** patients versus 0.7% in the control group, and there were significantly more withdrawals in the Vioxx group for causes including **hypertension, edema, hepatotoxicity, heart failure**, or **pathological laboratory findings**. The mean increases in systolic and diastolic blood pressure in the Vioxx group were 4.6 mmHg and 1.7 mmHg respectively, compared to 1.0 and 0.1 mmHg in the control NSAID group. Therefore, the promise of better patient outcomes and lowered medical costs from use of COX-2 inhibitors may not be as great as previously hoped. [http://en.wikipedia.org/wiki/COX-2_selective_inhibitor]

The answer? You absolutely need to know what *causes* your disease and pain and address it by first withdrawing the offender (like the mercury, pesticides, glutamates) and then you need to provide healing nutrients - *Nature's Medicines.*

Nature's Medicines Work Without Harming

If only everyone would apply Nature's principles *first* – we would see a lot more healing than we do. When seeking out information about the cause of disease and what to do, in book after book, by authors who are "just people" or even supposedly authoritarians (doctors, scientists), you are told the "what", but not told anything more. For example: Ginkgo is good for the brain. That's the "what". Without knowing the why, where, when and how, we've all been left in the dark, and thus not motivated to take the herb.

In another example, year after year news stories come on television telling us we need to eat more broccoli or just more "veges" in general. People hear it, think, "I guess they're right", but are never really motivated to do the right thing. If people only knew that the simple recommendation to "eat more veges", especially *raw* vegetables, if they really followed it, could prevent them from ever suffering horrendous diseases and pain. If they truly knew this, they'd be more likely to do it. If the weight of the truth were to be accurately conveyed, it would be screamed at people, forced upon them, even made a law.

Okay, so we can't be screaming at people. Let's at least understand that the difference between man's medicines, and God's medicines is that God's medicines simply don't do *harm* while doing good. Remember, man's medicines may indeed go to the problem, but can then go anywhere and everywhere else as well, causing harm in the places they are not supposed to go. But God's medicines *miraculously* concentrate where they do their good work, and if they go anywhere else, they only do *good.*

Another amazing property of ginkgo biloba is that ginkgo has an affinity for affecting brain tissues **more than other body tissues.** This is another reason ginkgo biloba and GbE is so promising for treating tinnitus and other brain, memory, and aging related conditions such as Alzheimer's disease. [http://www.tinnitus-treatment. info/treat-tinnitus-with-ginkgo-biloba/]

In spite of anything you may have ever heard about herbs (or any nutritional product, for that matter) there has *never* been any deaths or permanent harm from them (the only harm has been from improper handling/manufacturing, by other countries, such as when Japan introduced a toxin into tryptophan (an amino acid) in the manufacturing process). But compare this to the *hundreds* of people who die every *day* from drugs!

Drugs Often Don't Work

The statistics say that the leading cause of death in the United States, by far, is from tobacco – about 400,000 annually (and likely more from diseases caused by the tobacco that we're not brilliant enough, yet, to associate with tobacco). The statistics also say that about one-tenth that many, or 40,000 people die annually from an "adverse" reaction to a prescription or over-the-counter drug (especially pain killers like Tylenol!). What the statistics don't say is that the number of people dying from drugs is more likely *ten times higher* and thus causes deaths right up there with tobacco. The reason this is so, is because many people have died from, for example, kidney disease, and "kidney disease" is listed on their death certificate. What is not made clear is that *analgesic nephropathy* is a common reason for kidney disease (nephro = kidney, pathy = disease). So what killed them, analgesics or "kidney disease"? Well, the answer is that the drugs killed them. Pain killers, like acetaminophen (Tylenol) will slowly destroy a person's kidneys. However, when a death isn't instantaneous (like a car accident) nor obvious (like a cancerous tumor) the true underlying cause can often be missed.

Another example would be cholesterol-lowering drugs. Thousands of people are crying out for help on the internet saying that their "Lipitor" (a statin drug) is causing muscle weakness, cramping, and possibly their Parkinson's and other neurological diseases (note that these are the symptoms the drug manufacturer says are *rare*). The patients know that Lipitor is the culprit, but because the "cause and effect" is done over time, the statistics simply don't report the connection.

Peter H Langsjoen, MD, a specialist in congestive heart failure, wrote an article called "Statin-induced cardiomyopathy" in July, 2002. In it he said that the medical profession, for more than 30 years, have successfully created propaganda which has created a phony disease they call "hypercholesterolemia". He talks about the medical profession's dismal failure to cure this "disease" using their low fat diets and cholesterol-lowering drugs. He goes on to say that statins block the body's ability to make cholesterol, but that statins kill people – lots of people. He rightfully states that all patients taking statins become depleted in Coenzyme Q10, which eventually leads to heart failure after making the person suffer with fatigue, muscle weakness and soreness. Is he alone in this view? Hardly. Here are just a few titles of articles, by other scientists and doctors that can be found at: http://home.earthlink.net/~mbabco/statinlink.html

1. Paul Rosch, "Converting Millions Of Healthy People Into Perpetual Patients"
2. Maryann Napoli, "Cholesterol Skeptics And The Bad News About Statin Drugs"
3. Duane Graveline, M.D., M.P.H., "Transient Global Amnesia Associated With The Statin Drugs"
4. Joseph Mercola, M.D., "The Baycol Recall: How Safe is Your Statin?"

So why are doctors still prescribing, and why are patients still taking statins? Could the fact that billions are lost when a drug doesn't get prescribed have anything to do with it? Unfortunately, most doctors don't go home and read study after study to keep up on the truth. As a doctor friend once said to me, "*Most* doctors go home and take their wives to the opera or go out to dinner".

But statins aren't the only drug causing more harm than good. The truth is, there are many injuries and deaths that nobody even knows about, from many drugs. This is because there are people who have horrendous reactions to drugs who never go to a doctor about it. I have had many such reactions myself. Nobody knows but me – so I'm not in the statistics. If I were to die from long-term use of any medication, no-one would ever report it as a reaction to any drug. So you can see how I *know* that probably half a million or more people per year die from drug-related damage to their body. Back to the beauty of Nature's medicines.

Back To Nature

If you've read the entire book, you know that the mitochondria is the "energy" portion of your cells and is badly damaged by mercury.

ATP is the molecule that energizes the mitochondria. Damaged mito-chondria means a damaged brain and body.

> A large body of data emphasizes the central role of mitochondrial dysfunction during aging and as an early event in **neurodegenera-tive diseases**. As markers for the function of mitochondria, ATP levels and mitochondrial membrane potential were measured. The single components of **ginkgo biloba** [EGb 761] showed in both cell models **protection of the mitochondrial membrane** poten-tial...[*Pharmacol Res.* 2007 Dec;56(6):493-502.]

The Department of Psychiatry, School of Medicine, University of Mostar in Bosnia pleads in one study, with regard to the use of natural medicines, such as ginkgo:

> The aim is to encourage thinking about the meaning of natural medicines in the treatment of mental disorders and an attempt of preventing to push them (natural medicines) out totally into silence...[*Psychiatri Danub* 2007 Sep;19(3):241-4]

Doctors and scientists alike have witnessed millions of miracles with natural "medicines" like ginkgo, but don't pursue that avenue, mostly because it wouldn't profit them, nor the pharmaceutical indus-try, if people treated themselves by buying their "medicines" at the healthfood store.

What follows are 14 of what I consider to be the most important things you can do as a person with a brain and body damaged by mercury.

1 - Above All In Importance Is To Ingest Copious Quantities Of Phytochemicals

Phytochemicals are why mom told you to eat your vegetables. What mom didn't tell you, and didn't know, is that for optimum health, your diet really should consist *mostly* of plant foods (organ-ic, of course – i.e., *no pesticides*). But if you're sick and want to truly heal, your diet should consist 100% of plant foods, *mostly or all raw.*

Anything you eat that isn't a pure, fresh, whole, organic plant food can be *contrary* to optimum health, and is often something your body is merely forced to *deal* with not *heal* with. In eating meats, for example, you get undesirable fats and uric acid. Meat is a difficult-to-move fiberless mass going through the digestive tract. Meats leave an "acid ash" requiring the use of the body's calcium to neutralize those acids, causing calcium loss in bones and tissues. There are little to no protective nutrients in meats, and any that may have been there in the raw state, are destroyed by cooking. Can you ever eat meat? See "If You're Going To Cheat" in Chapter 12.

Regarding Organic Plant Foods As I discussed in Chapter 3, My husband and I eat at a popular salad bar restaurant in Southern California called "Souplantation". Because it is convenient to eat there once or twice a week (for example on very busy days) I was very concerned as to whether we were consuming pesticides – certainly something that would be contrary to our mission of healing and health maintenance I spent many months trying to find a lab that would test an organic salad vs. a "Souplantation" salad for me. Most labs declined, saying they only tested for the government, or for "commercial" entities. One told me I couldn't afford their fee (I believe he said $2,000!). Finally, in December, 2008, I found a wonderful lab, EMA, in California, that didn't hesitate to take my zip-lock bag of organic salad vs. "Souplantation" salad. Their fee was about one-fourth that which was previously quoted. The lab didn't know which salad was which, I'd labeled them "A" and "B". The results were that they found the salads to be nearly identical, and both essentially without pesticides.

Of the 159 pesticides and herbicides they tested for, only the "Souplantation" salad, had a barely detectible amount of "Chlorpyrifos" also known as Dursban. I wondered if it was because they washed their produce before serving, and could be washing off any residual pesticides making it safe for health-seekers to eat there. Unfortunately, I worked for many years in restaurants, and witnessed firsthand how food preparers would take a head of lettuce out of the large box containing many heads of lettuce, delivered by the quantity food companies, and plop that lettuce up on the cutting board without so much as a rinse. I *know* this practice goes on all over the world.

Souplantation is perhaps among the highest quality "salad bar" restaurants in the United States, easily judged by their obvious cleanliness and freshness of food – as well as the number of patrons that visit there daily, judging by the continuously filled tables in the dining room. I'm sure that is part of why we got the results we did. But a call to EMA lab director, David Elliott, also taught me that there are a possible 1,000 or so chemicals that could be used, and they only tested for about 159. He said that you can't wash many of them off (he scoffs at the soaps and vinegar vegetable washes people purchase – he said they don't work). He told me that some pesticides are "systemic" (taken up by the plant) and so, of course, cannot be washed off. Others are designed to "cling" to the plant and *not* wash off. But he also said that the worst pesticides are no longer allowed in the United States. Some of our food is imported, however.

For the second edition of this book I hope to get fruit from Costco tested. On the boxes of their beautiful-looking fruits are lists of the various pesticides, fungicides and herbicides used on the fruit. When I walk in that area of Costco I can *smell* the chemicals. What a difference in smell from Costco's produce section (smells of chemicals) to the organic farm stand across the street from my home (smells of fresh tomatoes and greens).

So the conclusion is to always be on the cautious side and choose organic for all your foods at home. Organic produce is mostly about avoiding pesticides, but it has been tested to be higher in nutrients as well.

Phytochemicals

In fact, there are many thousands of known and named protective nutrients, such as the aforementioned over 6,000 named polyphenols (just one category of phytochemicals) to date. Plant foods include vegetables (including starchy vegetables like corn), herbs, fruits, nuts and seeds, whole grains and beans. (Again, for people with cancer, immune problems, and viral problems, nuts, seeds and even grains, while rich in phytochemicals, are also extraordinarily high in the amino acid arginine - precursor to nitric oxide, and stimulus to viral and cancer cell growth - and are thus a major problem as also explained previously).

Scientists, studying phytochemicals continuously around the world, have discovered that these polyphenols are miraculously protective of the human body's 10-100 trillion cells, protecting them from cancer, viral attack, heavy metal attack and more. It seems we're always hearing new words, especially in "breaking news", that are **phytochemicals** (compounds in plants) of which polyphenols are the predominant antioxidants. Phytochemicals are all **"phenolic compounds"** and include monophenols like **apiole** in parsley, or **carnosol** in rosemary, or **carvacrol** in oregano and thyme. Then there are the flavonoids (those polyphenols) like the *flavonols* **quercetin** for example, in onions, tea, wine, apples and beans. There is **gingerol** from ginger (a *powerful* antiinflammatory). There is **kaempferol** in strawberries, cranberries, peas and more. There is **myricetin** in grapes, walnuts and more. There is **resveratrol** in grape skins (and of course, wine). There is **rutin** in citrus fruits and buckwheat and more. Also under the category of flavonoids are the *flavanones* like **hesperidin** as well as **naringenin** in citrus fruits. The herb milk thistle contains the flavanone **silybin** which is a powerful antioxidant targeting the liver. In fact, when two groups of animals were given poisonous mushrooms, the group also given silybin survived unscathed, while the group not given silybin *died*. Wow!

Also under the category of flavonoids are the *flavones*. There are many, but perhaps you've heard of **luteolin**. News reports have told us this antioxidant protects us against cancer among other things. The highest dietary sources of luteolin are celery, green peppers and camomile tea. Have you consumed any of those today?

In an attempt to identify **phytochemicals** contributing to the well-documented preventive effect of **plant-based diets** on **cancer** incidence **and mortality**, we have previously shown that certain **flavonoids** inhibit *in vitro* angiogenesis. Here, we show that the **flavonoid luteolin** inhibited tumor growth and angiogenesis in a murine xenograft model. [*Cancer Research* 64, 7936-7946, November 1, 2004]

Moving on, we have another category of flavonoids called *flavan-3-ols* (these names are all derived from how the molecules are put together).

Within this category are many well-known phytochemicals. One category of flavan-3-ols are **catechins** which are found in white and green tea, grapes, wine, apple juice, cocoa, lentils, and black-eyed peas. I ask you again, are you consuming copious quantities of these? You *cannot* hope to get all the protective phytochemicals you need from "supplements".

Also in the flavan-3-ols category is **epigallocatechin gallate,** which is also called EGCG, and is the miraculous molecule concentrated in green tea that lowers nitric oxide levels (antiinflammatory), helps a person lose weight, and is also protective against cancer.

There are many other flavan-3-ols. In fact, there are so many other phytochemicals, an entire encyclopedia of books could be written. So what's the answer? I think you know: Eat your fresh, pure, whole, fruits, vegetables, only whole unaltered grains, as well as raw nuts and seeds (if you don't have a viral or cancer problem already). God put all the protection you need into them. And don't worry about protein, all the amino acids (building blocks of protein) that you need are also in plant foods when you eat them whole and in abundance. Where do you think cows and horses get protein for those massive bodies and muscles? From plants!

Below is a good, but not complete list (we're discovering new things every day) of the major categories of phytochemicals. I found that studying this type of list is fascinating for the following reason. It seems that every day there's a report in the media about some fabulous antioxidant, as if we all need to run out to the healthstore and buy that one nutrient in a bottle or we won't be optimally healthy. With this list, when you hear of just such a "new" discovery, you can place it within the "plant kingdom", and know that the point is *not* that you need to run out and buy another expensive supplement (though taking some supplements to target areas of damage and to help your body heal better and faster is a great idea) — but to make sure your diet is made up literally *entirely* of pure, fresh, whole, organic plant foods of all types. In this way you will not only be consuming the more than 6,000 known phenolic compounds (only one of the seven categories of phytochemicals below), but the many thousands more compounds God saw fit to put in plant foods to keep you healthy.

Why mostly raw? Because many if not most antioxidant compounds are destroyed by heat, air and light, so cooking a food will render them useless. I often use the cooked pea vs. raw pea example. Put the raw pea in the ground and it will grow. Put a cooked pea in the ground – it will rot.

In addition, we can palatably and enjoyably eat raw plant foods – while we don't *usually* eat raw meats or eggs. In each category I give just one (there are many) examples of a food you could eat to obtain that God-given phytochemical. Some of the phytochemicals are in plants we don't eat (like mistletoe) and put there by Nature, obviously for other reasons (like the health of the plant itself, or of animals that consume the plant).

PHYTOCHEMICALS *Plant Nutrients – Powerful Antioxidants and Protectors*
PHENOLIC COMPOUNDS
<u>Monophenols</u>

    Apiole – parsley
    Carnosol – rosemary
    Carvacrol – oregano
    Dillapiole – dill
    Rosemarinol - rosemary

<u>Flavonoids (polyphenols)</u> *red, blue, purple pigments*
    Flavanols
        Quercetin – onions
        Gingerol – ginger
        Kaempferol – strawberries
        Myricetin – grapes
        Resveratrol – grapes
        Rutin – citrus fruits
        Isorhamnetin - mustard
    Flavanones
        Hesperidin – oranges
        Naringenin – grapefruit
        Silybin – milk thistle herb
        Eriodictyol - lemons

Flavones
    Apigenin – celery
    Tangeritin – tangerine
    Luteolin – green peppers
Flavan-3-ols
    Catechins – green tea and many foods
    There are many subcategories in this category such
    as Epigallocatechin gallate (EGCG) and Theaflavin
    from black tea and many foods
Anthocyanins (flavonals) – *red, purple or blue fruits and
vegetables*
        Pelargonidin – raspberry
        Peonidin – cherry
        Cyanidin – red pears
        Delphinidin – bilberry
        Malvidin – blueberry
        Petunidin – blueberries and purple grapes
    Isoflavones (phytoestrogens)
        Daidzein – chickpeas
        Genistein – legumes
        Glycitein – soy
    Coumestans (phytoestrogens) – various herbs
    Coumestrol – brussels sprouts
Phenolic Acids
        Ellagic acid – walnuts
        Gallic acid – mango
        Salicyclic acid – wheat
        Tannic acid – berries
        Vanillin – vanilla beans
        Capsaicin – chili peppers
        Curcumin - turmeric
Hydroxycinnamic Acids
        Caffeic acid – artichoke
        Chlorogenic acid – pineapple
        Cinnamic acid – aloe
        Ferulic acid – oats
        Coumarin - corn

Lignans (phytoestrogens)
  Silymarin – milk thistle
  Matairesinol – broccoli
  Secoisolariciresinol – seeds, carrots
  Pinoresinol and lariciresinol – sesame seed
Tyrosol esters
  Tyrosol – olive oil
  Hydroxytyrosol – olive oil
  Oleocanthal – olive oil
  Oleuropein – olive oil
Stilbenoids
  Resveratrol – grapes
  Pterostilbene – blueberries
  Piceatannol - grapes

TERPENES (ISOPRENOIDS)

Carotenoids (tetraterpenoids)
  Carotene – *orange pigments*
  Lycopene - tomatoes
  Neurosporene - tomatoes
  Phytofluene – algae foods
  Phytoene – algae foods
  Xanthophylls – *yellow pigments*
  Cryptoxanthin – red bell peppers
  Zeaxanthin – sweet yellow corn
  Astaxanthin – microalgae and yeast
  Lutein – kale, spinach, romaine lettuce
Monoterpenes
  Limonene – oils of citrus, cherries, various herbs
  Perillyl alcohol – citrus oils, various herbs
Saponins - legumes
Lipids
  Phytosterols – nuts, seeds, beans, grains, corn
    Campesterol – buckwheat
    Beta sitosterol – avocadoes, some nuts, seeds, grains
    Gamma sitosterol – soybeans

Stigmasterol – buckwheat
Tocopherols – vitamin E
Omega-3,6,9 fatty acids – dark green leafy vegeta
bles, grains, legumes, nuts
    Gamma-linolenic acid – evening primrose, bor
age, black currant
Triterpenoid
    Oleanolic acid – various herbs, garlic, cloves
    Ursolic acid – various fruits and herbs like apples
and cranberries, peppermint and prunes
    Betulinic acid – various plants not commonly eaten
    Moronic acid – Brazilian propolis (from bees)

BETALAINS
Betalains
    Betacyanins
        Betanin – beets
        Isobetanin – beets
        Probetanin – beets
        Neobetanin – beets
    Betaxanthins (non glycosidic versions)
        Indicaxanthin – beets
        Vulgaxanthin - beets

ORGANOSULFIDES
Dithioltiones (isothiocyanates)
    Sulphoraphane – cabbage
Thiosulphonates (allium compounds)
    Allyl methyl trisulfide – garlic and onions
    Diallyl sulfide – garlic and onions

INDOLES, GLUCOSINOLATES
Indole-3-carbinol – mustard greens
Sulforophane – broccoli
3,3'Diindolylmethane (DIM) - broccoli
Sinigrin – broccoli
Allicin – garlic
Alliin – garlic
Allyl isothiocyanate – horseradish

Piperine – black pepper
Syn-propanethial-S-oxide - onions
PROTEIN INHIBITORS
Protease inhibitors - legumes
OTHER ORGANIC ACIDS
Oxalic acid – spinach
Phytic acid (inositol hexaphosphate) seeds
Tartaric acid – apricots
Anacardic acid - cashews

This list is not complete – indeed, over 6,000 polyphenols alone have been named! But, if you find that a new nutrient is on this list, and you are consuming a diet rich or entirely of pure, fresh, whole, organic plant foods, you are likely getting the nutrient already. If the new "discovery" isn't on the list, the category to which it belongs likely will be, and that would be information enough to discern whether you need to supplement, or already get it in your diet. For me, the list serves as a powerful reminder as to how imporant it is for our diet to be made up of plant foods – because we simply cannot get the protective nutrients God meant for us to have any other way.

Of course this list of phytochemicals doesn't mention the dozens of other needed nutrients, like amino acids, vitamins, macro minerals and trace minerals. But these are also there in the plant foods right along with the polyphenols and such. So again no worries, if your diet is made up almost entirely of pure, fresh, whole, organic plant foods, you will get everything you need, and nothing that you don't.

Raw Is Essential There is absolutely nothing wrong with consuming a meal of cooked foods, but as a person seeking true *healing*, let's make sure we thoroughly understand the truth. The truth is, when you cook fresh fruits and vegetables, much of what makes them so wonderful (all those phytochemicals) are *destroyed*. A study using temperatures far lower (under 200°) than what you normally use to cook food discovered that 50% of the phytochemical activity was destroyed. [Larrauri J.A. et al. Effect of drying temperature on the stability of polyphenols and antioxidant activity of red grape pomace peels. *Journal of Agricultural and Food Chemistry* 1997, vol. 45, no. 4, pp. 1390-1393]

When you cook your fresh fruits and vegetables in hot oil or in an oven, or for long periods of time on the stove, you destroy the anti-oxidants nearly if not completely. Your body needs "living" foods. I've been saying for decades that raw is best. Since the 1980's every time a report would come out about how healthful and cancer-preventive vegetables or fruits are, I would tell family, friends and co-workers, "but they have to be raw". Now, in November, 2008, comes a study, reported at the American Association for Cancer Research's Seventh Annual International Conference on Frontiers in Cancer Prevention Research. This the first time I've seen where raw vs cooked was studied and reported upon. Hallelujah! Better late than never!

Among smokers, the protective effect of cruciferous vegetable intake ranged from a 20 percent reduction in risk to a 55 percent reduction in risk depending on the type of vegetable consumed and the duration and intensity of smoking. For example, among current smokers, only the consumption of **raw cruciferous vegetables** was associated with risk reduction of lung cancer. [Lead author Li Tang, Ph.D., a post-doctoral fellow at Roswell Park Cancer Institute]

2 - "Wait/See" Give Your Body A Chance To Heal

August, 2008, the big news is that there is a new recommendation for testing for prostate cancer. The news is:

An independent panel of experts today recommended **against** prostate cancer screenings for men older than 74 and advised younger men to weigh the potential benefits and risks before undergoing the prostate screening test. [http://abcnews.go.com/WN/story?id=5513560&page=1]

They go on to say that prostate cancer is the second leading cause of cancer death in males after lung cancer. However, screening for prostate cancer, especially in men over 70 is unlikely to benefit them because it's a slow-growing cancer, and old age is more likely to cause the death of the individual than prostate cancer. In addition, there is a problem with a false-positive test leading to unnecessary and death-hastening treatments! Even screening to "catch the cancer early" has not proven to reduce any chance of dying from the disease.

Well, folks, I'm here to tell you that this same recommendation applies to nearly all medical testing. I know personally, because I've undergone thousands and thousands of dollars worth of testing for *absolutely* nothing. If you find this difficult to believe, take your own survey. Ask everybody you meet how many medical tests they have had, and how many of those tests discovered the *cause* of their problem.

Sadly, most people may not grasp the truth in this until they've undergone thousands and thousands of dollars worth of testing, with no definitive answer as to the cause of their disease. Often it takes a lifetime of searching and not finding to realize the error in it all – and then you can't go back and do it over. Apply this scenario to millions of people every year. Perhaps you went to the doctor because of chronic pain. People by the hundreds of thousands are sent home to suffer for months more until they again go to their doctors for help, and he/she thinks of another test to do. Often that test will also come back "negative".

One doctor I worked for years ago told me that the reason many tests come back negative, or "within range", and thus don't tell doctors anything are two-fold. First is that the doctor isn't doing the right tests (for example, if he's testing for mercury, it won't be found in the blood test he's doing, but must be captured in the urine after the patient takes a provoking agent, hence, his test comes back "negative"). The second reason doctors rarely find anything until it's "late" or "too late" even, is that their tests aren't sensitive enough. My doctor friend told me that many diseases that cause symptoms and pain don't yet show up on the "insensitive" tests doctors routinely used. For example, I had a girlfriend, in her 30's, who was extremely anxiety-ridden to the point of being unable to hold down a job. A routine blood test she had when the symptoms first began showed that her thyroid was a bit out of whack, but the doctor didn't think much about it. Time went by, and her anxiety got to the point of panic on a daily basis, and by this time, her thyroid reading was off the charts, but it was too late – it hadn't been caught early enough (or apparently the doctor hadn't been able to grasp the significance of the earlier testing) and she was found dead in her home, keys in hand. She was trying to take herself to the doctor.

Then, when I was in my early 50's when I couldn't breathe, I felt fatigued beyond fatigued and had "lupus-like" symptoms in my joints and such, I went to a doctor. She did extensive testing. I paid out my thousands again. Apparently it was found that I had excessively clumped red blood cells and so she suspected something (although she didn't tell me what) for which she sent me to the hospital for an arterial blood gas test (a painful puncture of your artery to withdraw blood). The test came back normal, so I didn't have the deadly disease she suspected (I discovered she was looking for polycythemia). Even though I still couldn't breathe and I still felt like death warmed over and my joints ached and more…...*she didn't have a clue what to do next.* She "fired me". Told me I "might be better served by a different doctor". Again, so much time and money spent, without results, and no help at all for the suffering.

Folks, and if you're a doctor I'm sorry, but it's true, *doctors just don't have all the answers.* Consider this: If a doctor finds you have a tumorous cancer, he can "cut it out" and give you toxic drugs. But (and here's where I really need you to use your power of reasoning): He can't **stop** *more tumors from growing elsewhere.* You can't apply highly toxic chemicals to a body already so toxic it succumbed to cancer, and truly believe this is how you stop cancer forever. Indeed! Is he going to just keep poisoning and cutting until there's nothing left of you? And *why* is it that we subject ourselves to this? Is it because when we go to the doctor it is foremost in our minds that he has had years and years of training, and years and years of "experience", and he wears a white lab coat, and his office smells sterile, and he has a wall of impressive looking books and diplomas, and there are other people running around the office in scrubs and white coats, and they greet you at the counter as if they are totally in control? After all, they take your insurance card and reassure you that your visit and treatments will be "billed" – not to worry, you'll have little or no "out of pocket" expense. Your decisions are made for you – you don't even have to think. Good thing, too, because you've got your illness on your mind.

On the opposite side of the coin is if you decide to go the "alternative", "holistic" or "nutritional" route. With that decision *you're on your own.* There are no people in white lab coats hustling and bustling around you taking your insurance card reassuring you "it will all be paid for". You are not only 100% responsible for finding out what is causing your disease and what is best to do for it....but you're completely on your own to *do* it, and pay for it. There will be nobody squeezing wheatgrass juice for you when you're too sick and weak to do it yourself. And if that's not bad enough, there will be naysayers, scoffers and people who tell you you're crazy.

Your God-Given Internal, Multi-Faceted, Marvelous And Often Miraculous System Of Healing And Rebuilding

So what's the answer? The answer is that you were born with a God-given internal, multi-faceted, marvelous and often miraculous system of healing and rebuilding. Indeed, man didn't even appreciate fully just one of his internal systems called "stem cells" until just this century! It was in about the year 2000 that man's attention turned away from his microscope and the debate about embryonic stem cells (as if embryos were the only source of stem cells) and onto the many other sources, including bone marrow and even your own fat cells. That's right! You have many, many sources of stem cells which God put within you to continually *repair* what gets damaged. Yes, it was in about the year 2000 that a major lightbulb began to shine on the field of stem cells and we now know that your stem cells exist and work in your body *throughout your entire life.*

Along with this realization has surged the field of "regenerative medicine" wherein many are now beginning to *truly* realize that your own body can heal, if protected from the pollutants (toxins) causing disease, and empowered with the various natural modalities that give the body a chance to heal. So, if you don't cut, burn or poison yourself to death first....even if it takes years and years, your very best opportunity to heal is found within your own body, and within God's kingdom of pure, whole foods, herbs, sunshine, activity, sweating, oxygen and similar. It took me about 11 years to see the last lymph gland shrink back down to normal after being diagnosed with lymphoma and embarking upon 100% natural modalities to heal myself. But I lived my life all those years, going to school, marrying, even having children! Quite a different scenario from someone with cancer that embarks upon chemo, radiation and surgery! But most of all...quite a different *outcome*. I was in my late 20's when I was diagnosed...I'm 55 now.

3 - Stop Consuming Bad Fats

Unfortunately getting the "good fats" into your body isn't as easy as simply adding a supplement containing "essential fatty acids" (like the popular 'fish oils') while continuing to consume altered, heated, oxidized, saturated, hydrogenated, and trans fats! Looking at it from man's point of view is complex and very confusing. Looking at it from God's point of view is simple. Fats in Nature are protected and must be pure (not from sources tainted with mercury). Nuts are in heavy shells, protecting them from sun, air, light, heat. The heavy shells protect the fatty acids from oxidizing and becoming free radicals (bad fats). Avocadoes are covered by a thick peel. This protects the fats so that when you consume the avocado, you are getting healthful fatty acids, not harmful. So if you consume *only* fats like these you're doing the most healthful, protective and repairative thing for your body. Studies clearly show that when you consume a bad fat along with a good fat, the bad fat "wins" the race to your cells.

So bad fats are bullies. Here is a "nutrition made easy" primer. I know that many people, especially young people with nothing major wrong, can't understand how something that goes into the mouth has any effect whatsoever on parts of their body distant from their mouth! Well, it works like this: Your body is made up of some 10 to 100 trillion cells (the scientists can't give us an exact number). But whether 10 or 100 trillion *that's a LOT of cells.* Each cell is a living entity in itself. The outer cell membrane is the "skin" of the cell which works to allow *into* the cell only beneficial substances, and keep *out* of the cell, harmful substances. There are also "receptor sites" all over the cell surface that accept molecules and atoms of substances that they are suppose to "work" with. For example, on every cell are numerous receptor sites for vitamin C. If you don't have enough vitamin C, a glucose molecule can take up that site.

The health of each of your cells translates into the health of your entire body. If your cells do not have healthy cell membranes, or the cell membranes are damaged, very harmful substances can enter, causing the cell to mutate, replicate wildly out of control, and even die. When you have millions of cells mutating, you have "genetic" diseases. When you have millions of cells replicating wildly, you have cancer. When you have millions of cells dying, you have things like kidney failure, liver failure, or heart failure...or even death of the entire "organism" – you.

However, if each cell membrane is made up of the essential fatty acids, phospholipids, unoxidized cholesterol and proteins as Nature designed, those cells will have the optimum chance of doing the job of keeping your cells (you) healthy. If all the trace minerals, bio-flavonoids, vitamins and other molecules designed by your Creator to protect your cells are there, standing guard at your cells, or occupying their receptor sites, then they will, again, have the optimum chance of doing the job of keeping your cells (you) healthy. The ideal scenario then would mean you would live without disease, pain and suffering, and with optimum strength to live, accomplish and enjoy life!

Here's an analogy. Imagine a construction worker showing up at the job site to build a home. But when he/she gets there, there are no plans, no bricks, no wood, no tools. Also there is no protective fence around the site. Along come some "bad guys"....they attack the construction worker. Having no tools, no machinery, nothing to protect himself nor hide behind, he is defenseless, and the bad guys beat him up and leave him for dead. That construction worker is like a defenseless cell. The "bad guys" are like bad fats and toxins.

This is like a body filled with chips, beer, "fast foods", high levels of glutamates from "Top Ramen", canned soups and commercial salad dressings. The cells are not being given all the nutrients they need to withstand the "bad guys" and at the same time the body is being filled with "bad guys" in the way of oxidized fats (free radicals), gluta-mates, sugar, chemical food additives, etc. A body can only withstand this for a number of years before cells can no longer stand up under the onslaught. Something as toxic as mercury hastens the damage with lightening speed both as a direct free radical "catalyzer" and by doing damage to any protective systems that exist within the body.

To keep the bad guys from being bullies, you simply must stop consuming foods that are full of "bad guys", i.e., oxidized and altered fat molecules. When you eat "junk" all day, taking even hands full of supplements, or thinking you're erasing the bad by eating a carrot and an apple every day, is like trying to bail out the sinking Titanic with a teaspoon.

Again, studies show overwhelmingly that when you eat bad fats (saturated, heated, oxidized, processed, trans, hydrogenated) even if you eat good fats (unoxidized, omega-3, unsaturated, mono) the bad fats are bullies and knock the good guys aside to take their place on your cells and elsewhere. Only good fats build healthy cell membranes and hormones, and yet the typical American diet is mostly, if not all, bad fats.

The study quoted below is saying that when you consume veg-etable fats as found in bottles of processed oils, "sunflower oil", "saf-flower oil", fast foods, etc. (LA = linolenic acid, Omega-6), even if you also consume "fish oils", "flax oil", etc. (ALA = alpha-linolenic acid, Omega-3), the LA overrides any benefit the ALA might offer. Most people either consume *no* ALA/Omega-3, or only consume damaged, oxidized Omega-3 along with mercury when they eat fish thinking they're doing a good thing. Nevertheless, no matter how much ALA/Omega-3 you consume, if you also eat processed "vege-table oils" you render the good fatty acids ineffective. The body needs to convert ALA to enough EPA (eicosapentaenoic acid – the "ver-sion" of Omega-3 that does miraculous and healthful things for your body's heart, antiinflammatory, hormones), but LA gets in the way. At the same time AA (arachidonic acid – the *inflammatory* fatty acid as found in meats and dairy) is increased by consumption of LA.

...regardless of high ALA (omega-3), high dietary LA (omega-6) (11.6% LA and 1.2% ALA) decreased EPA (the antiinflammatory fatty acid desired when consuming fish oils, for example) and led to a high heart membrane AA (arachidonic acid – inflammatory), and Ca(2+)-dependent cPLA(2) with a marked increase in nitrosative stress (there's nitric oxide again!). Our results suggest that the potential cardiovascular benefit of ALA is achieved only when dietary LA is reduced concomitantly rather than fed with high LA diet. [*Am J Physiol Heart Circ Physiol* 2007 Nov;293(5):H2919-27.]

4 - Fight Inflammation By Removing The Cause And Using Nature's Antiinflammatories

Psoriasis, migraines, and multiple sclerosis as well as many if not all diseases, have inflammation as the component that precedes cell damage, as well as accounts for the pain of the disease. Inflammation is the body's *response* to attack and damage.

To protect your body, you *must* consume copious quantities of raw plant foods which contain *bioactive* compounds. Inflammation is only the *beginning*. For example, it may start with migraines but can go on to even far worse diseases. The optimal way to fight inflammation is by minimizing exposure to toxic substances while providing your body with copious quantities of phytochemicals.

"Malignant cells are characterized by alterations in multiple signaling pathways that promote proliferation, inhibit apoptosis, promote angiogenesis in the case of solid tumors, and enable cancer cells to invade and migrate through tissues. **A variety of foods and their bioactive dietary constituents** appear to have merit in reducing cancer risk and modifying tumor behavior." [Davis CD, Milner JA. *Curr Cancer Drug Targets.* 2007 Aug;7(5):410-5.]

The researchers in the text box above are saying that cancer is caused because of alterations in our cells. Cancer isn't the *beginning* of a disease process, it is the *end*. Cancer is usually a lengthy process, and starts years before the person knows they have cancer. Cancer starts with attack upon unprotected cells (phytochemicals are what protect your cells), then cells go through a "response" phase while they are still somewhat strong, which includes glutamate release, nitric oxide excess, CGRP release, inflammation etc., and *then* as they become weak (and especially with the continued assault of toxins, and without the help of those phytochemicals) aberrancies and proliferation of cells occur, i.e., cancer or death.

We now know that deadly gases, plastics, and metals have been proven to cause an alteration in cells. **Protection of cells is "dose dependent". If you are bombarded by a million toxic molecules, you could very likely survive if you have a million protective molecules standing guard.** The reason someone succumbs quickly to an intensely poisonous assault is because the number of toxic molecules were far greater than the number of protective molecules. This would be true nearly always if a person swallows any amount, for example, of lead or arsenic; or is unfortunate enough to be near a radiation disaster (like Russia's Chernobyl disaster).

There are toxins we consume daily without even knowing it (like plastics) that interfere with normal hormone processes. Did you know, for example that PCB in plastic "demasculinates"? PCBs are anti-androgenous - meaning "against" the male hormone. It is something to think seriously about as you learn about the many people who don't *feel* like the sex they were assigned at birth.

The only way to truly fight inflammation is by lowering the toxic load on the body first, then saturating the body with every phytochemical Nature gave us for protection.

5 - Antioxidants Stand Guard To Protect Your Cells

Nearly every natural substance from "A" to "zinc" has antioxidant properties. Of course this is by "grand design", because oxidation is the body's worst enemy. An antioxidant is a substance that protects your cells against oxidative damage – just like rusting. Consider what happens when you leave something out in the wind, rain and sunshine.

It will rust due to oxidative damage…and so do your cells. Only instead of being coated with "iron oxide" (rust) your cells, when bombarded by oxygen free radicals, degrade, explode, shrivel up, stop functioning, even die. The free radicals that oxidize your cells come from toxic metals, oxygen itself, oxidized (heated and processed) fats, toxic chemicals and more. So if you don't provide copious antioxidants to your body, you are exposing all 10-100 trillion of your body's cells to a battle they cannot win. Of course this means disease, chronic pain, horrific diagnoses from doctors – even early death.

The good news is that by far the richest source of anitoxidants are fresh, whole fruits and vegetables which contain all those phytochemicals. Among the phytochemicals are over 6,000 polyphenols (the most studied of all phytochemicals). Phyto (plant) chemicals not only give fruits and vegetables their color, but also provide enormous health benefits due to all phytochemicals' anti-inflammatory and anti-oxidative actions. In addition, phytochemicals also activate the key enzyme (AMP kinase) that helps restore cellular ATP levels (damaged by mercury). ATP is the molecule that sparks the energy in your cells. Without energy, the cell cannot do its job, and even dies.

Indeed, the *only* hope of protecting your 10-100 trillion cells from being attacked and altered by chemicals is via a body *saturated* with antioxidants. It is beyond me as to why any intelligent person today would fail to make *sure* they consume a diet rich in pure, fresh, whole, (preferably organic) fruits and vegetables if they do *nothing* else.

Studies show that **high levels of carotenoids** and **vitamin C** seem to decrease the level of circulating high sensitivity **CRP** (hs-CRP). (My note: hs-CRP is one of the acute-phase proteins in inflammation found high in the blood when there is inflammation and damage somewhere in the body, such as found in cancer, diabetes type 2, obesity, smoking and cardiovascular disease.) In addition, **high consumption of vegetables and fruit are associated with lower levels of circulating hs-CRP.** [Nanri A et al. Impact of C-reactive protein on disease risk and its relation to dietary factors. *Asian Pac J Cancer Prev* 2007 Apr-Jun;8(2):167-77.]

6 - Understand Inflammation

Inflammation is actually your body's response to a series of events all having to do with an attack upon your cells (by physical injury as well as pollutants and parasites). The damaged tissue then releases chemicals that attract white blood cells (which come to your defense and try to clean up damage). The white blood cells then attack the microorganisms (parasites) as well as consume damaged cells. During this entire process "**cytokines**" (hormone-like signalling molecules) are produced that increase inflammation because inflammation is actually used by the body in an attempt to heal. One cytokine called **IL-6** stimulates another chemical called **C-reactive protein**, which is a "biomarker" of inflammation.

When you read studies about scientists trying to stop inflammation (they are looking for either a drug or a phytochemical to stop the inflammation) you will read how they measured the "biomarkers of inflammation" as their way of proving whether their antiinflammatory compound was a success. CRP is a biomarker. You can ask your doctor for a CRP blood test. Oddly, doctors don't usually order this test except when they suspect you've had a heart attack.

When parasites attack weakened cells, the infection causes a release of cytokines (review above) to which your body responds by producing a protein complex called **NF-κB** which plays a key role in regulating the immune response to infection. The only reason I put these terms here is because when new "miracle foods", herbs or nutrients are discovered (or even drugs), you will hear or read how the miracle compound has a role in ameliorating any of the above processes, and thus inflammation, infection, cancer, etc. Doctors rarely explain any of this to you because they either don't know it themselves, or they believe you won't understand, or they don't want to take the time to explain. Many doctors for whom I've written articles and books, have told me to "dumb it down" (a term that has always bothered me) and not use all the "big words". So for those that care, I've written this here as a good place to start your own research and better understanding of your own disease process.

How do you fight inflammation? In addition to the right diet, you can take some supplements known to be powerful antioxidants and antiinflammatory. The good news is that you can "experiment" safely. *No-one* has been injured or died from taking a supplement that you will find on the shelf of your health store. No-one. Only once in my entire lifetime has this ever even been an issue, and that was when a Japanese manufacturer of L-tryptophan produced a tainted batch of the amino acid by using faulty manufacturing processes. As I've said before, compare this to the thousands upon thousands who die every year from drug damage. The latest statistics show that there are approximately 40,000 *known* deaths every year from prescription and over-the-counter drugs. Again, deaths from vitamins and herbs aren't even on the list, because they are non-existent. [Source: Mokdad, Ali H., PhD, James S. Marks, MD, MPH, Donna F. Stroup, PhD, MSc, Julie L. Gerberding, MD, MPH, "Actual Causes of Death in the United States, 2000," *Journal of the American Medical Association*, March 10, 2004, Vol. 291, No. 10, pp. 1238, 1241.]

I do make sure I know what each supplement is and does. I often start by *doubling* the recommended amount on the bottle once I've educated myself as to the phytochemical content, it's action in the body, and its application to my situation. For example, I've been taking "Red Clover Combination" for over 20 years (the formula includes cascara which aids intestinal peristalsis for elimination). I've found I can take as many as I need to do the job, which for me is normally about one with each meal (like the label says), but at other times, I might take three or four with each meal. Then there are times I don't take any for a while. You need to know what the supplement is and does, and adjust it to your own needs.

7 - Supplements That Suppress Nitric Oxide And Other Inflammatory Compounds

Turmeric [The Active Component Is Curcumin]
Turmeric is antiinflammatory. Studies show that it interferes with the NF-κB pathway spoken of above (one of the inflammatory mark-

ers brought about by parasitic infection) and thus it ameliorates inflammation. There are some who call the yellow pigment of turmeric (**curcumin**) the most miraculous of all herbal compounds because of its powerful antiinflammatory effects.

> Our data suggest that curcumin can inhibit P. gingivalis LPS-induced cytokine expression, and that this could be due to the inhibition of the NF-kappaB pathway [*Pharmacology* 2008 Oct 10;82(4):264-269.] It seems that curcumin attenuates acute lung injury probably through improving oxidative stress and **inhibiting NF-kappaB-mediated expression of inflammatory cytokines.** [*Eur Respir J* 2008 Sep 17.]

As an added "bonus", turmeric is hepatoprotective, meaning it protects your liver. Your liver is your largest and most important "detox" organ in the body (kidneys, skin, and lungs being next). When the liver is unable to do the job of detoxing, you're in trouble. As just one example of how important your liver is: Every year people get drunk, then take acetaminophen because they don't feel well, go to bed, and are found dead in the morning. Alcohol is so toxic to the liver, disabling it, so when you then take acetaminophen, your liver cannot "detox" the chemical, and it becomes deadly.

If you're thinking of doing one of those liver flushes that require you to drink olive oil and epsom salts, you may want to take turmeric instead. In studies with animals, the ones given arsenic were fully protected when also given curcumin. The same applied to other toxins and liver conditions in people and animals given turmeric (curcumin) along with the toxin.

Arsenic causes DNA damage by generating reactive oxygen species (my note: usually refers to nitric oxide) and enhancement of lipid peroxidation levels. **Curcumin** counteracted the damage by quenching the reactive oxygen species, decreasing the level of lipid peroxidation, and increasing the levels of phase II detoxification enzymes like catalase, superoxide dismutase (SOD), and glutathione peroxidase. Curcumin also elevated the level of polymerase, a repair enzyme. [Barbara Minton, Natural Health Editor, *Natural-News.com* Curcumin Tempers Arsenic Toxicity Through DNA Repair September 10, 2008 quoting the *Journal of Clinical Biochemistry and Nutrition.*]

To evaluate the ability of **Curcuma** longa (CL) and Tinospora cordifolia (TC) formulation to prevent anti-tuberculosis (TB) treatment (ATT) induced hepatotoxicity. The herbal formulation **prevented hepatotoxicity** significantly and improved the disease outcome as well as patient compliance without any toxicity or side effects. [*World J Gastroenterol.* 2008 Aug 14;14(30):4753-62]

Curcumin was effective in **preventing and reversing cirrhosis**, probably by its ability of reducing TGF-beta expression. These data suggest that curcumin might be an effective antifibrotic and fibrolitic drug in the treatment of chronic hepatic diseases. [*Fundam Clin Pharmacol* 2008 Aug;22(4):417-27]

According to a 2004 study published in the journal *Science*, curcumin fights genetic damage that causes cystic fibrosis in mice. In another study, rats genetically predisposed to multiple sclerosis developed few or no symptoms of this disease after being treated with turmeric. Curcumin also shows promise in protecting the liver from alcohol-induced damage. Turmeric is approved by German health officials as a treatment for dyspeptic disorders because it stimulates bile secretion from the gall bladder. And, the anti-inflammatory activity of turmeric root has been compared to topical hydrocortisone with equal efficacy.

I personally take two or three of a 400 mg *standardized* turmeric in vegetarian capsules (95% curcumin) several times daily. Standardized herbal extracts are concentrated extracts which have one or more of its ingredients at a "standard" level. This gives you a constant dose of that particular ingredient, in this case curcumin. Thus, we consumers can rely on the herb supplement to deliver a therapeutic dose of the component we are seeking.

EGCG

EGCG is Epigallocatechin Gallate, a compound found mostly in green tea. Taken as a supplement, EGCG has been shown in numerous studies to **suppress elevated levels of nitric oxide and nitric oxide synthase** (the enzyme responsible for turning the amino acid arginine + oxygen into nitric oxide). Suppressing excess nitric oxide is just "what the doctor ordered" (okay, so your doctor didn't order, but maybe he should!) to prevent migraines, inflammation, and body-wide damage from inflammation.

Nitric oxide does have "good guy, bad guy" properties, like so many other compounds necessary for life. Oxygen would be a great example. The right amount keeps you oxygenated and healthy…too much can cause brain damage! Mercury-damaged immune systems and glutamatergic systems, however, chronically produce too *much* nitric oxide. For these folks, taking the bottle's recommended daily amount is the key. But if any "flairs" in inflammation occur, EGCG might be used along with the other nitric-oxide lowering (antiinflammatory) supplements to hasten pain relief.

EGCG effectively mitigates cellular damage by lowering the inflammatory reaction and reducing the lipid peroxidation and **nitric oxide** generated radicals leading to the oxidative stress. [*Cardiovasc Hematol Disord Drug Targets* 2007 Jun;7(2):135-44.]

EGCG has stimulatory properties that help a person lose weight (thermogenic). If you are thin already, EGCG might not be for you. In addition, if you use caffeine as a vasoconstrictor, EGCG may prove too much for you as a supplement. As for me, I'm about 103 pounds soaking wet, so I don't use EGCG.

Ginger

Ginger is perhaps the most powerful anti-nitric oxide, antiinflammatory herb of all. You may have heard about ginger's powerful anti-nausea effect – able to even stop a person from vomiting. It's true. It's also completely safe, even during pregnancy. And one of the reasons ginger works so powerfully is because nitric oxide excess is involved in feeling nauseous.

This makes ginger one of the supplements of choice for migraineurs. Again, you must take enough. This usually means 3-4 capsules of the herb at a time. You may be limited by a burning in the stomach if you don't take ginger carefully. To take without food you can chew up eggshells to neutralize the stomach acid first, then the ginger can be taken with water. Otherwise, take ginger in the middle or towards the end of a snack or meal.

With this and *all* supplements, as someone who has a brain and body damaged by mercury, it is important to use only "V-caps" (vegetarian capsules) because the gelatin capsules are approximately 11% free glutamates! When you take many capsules daily, that 11% contributes a significant amount of free glutamates to a body that cannot handle *any*.

It is proposed that administration of **ginger** may exert abortive and prophylactic effects in migraine headache without any side-effects. [Mustafa T et al. Ginger (Zingiber officinale) in migraine headache. *J. Ethnopharmacol.* 1990 Jul;29(3):267-73.]

The present study suggests that zingerone (**Ginger**) has an efficient ONOO(-) (**nitric oxide**) scavenging ability, which may be a potent ONOO(-) scavenger for the protection of the cellular defense activity against ONOO(-)- involved diseases. [Shin SG et al. Zingerone as an antioxidant against peroxynitrite. *J Agric Food Chem.* 2005 Sep 21;53(19):7617-22.]

Our results indicate that [6]-**gingerol** is a **potent inhibitor of NO** synthesis and also an effective protector against peroxynitrite-mediated damage. [Ippoushi K et al. [6]-Gingerol inhibits nitric oxide synthesis in activated J774.1 mouse macrophages and prevents peroxynitrite-induced oxidation and nitration reactions. *Life Sci* 2003 Nov 14;73(26):3427-37.]

...**zingerone** [ginger], and **curcumin** [turmeric] significantly **inhibited the cellular production of proinflammatory mediators** such as TNF-alpha and **nitric oxide.** [Woo HM et al. *Life Sci* 2007 Feb 13;80(10):926-31.]

L-Lysine

Lysine is a single amino acid that is in opposition to arginine (also a single amino acid). Arginine is the direct building block for nitric oxide. So using lysine daily *along* with a diet lower in arginine than lysine is important for migraneurs and anyone with herpes or cancer. L-lysine has proven to be an effective agent for reduction of occurrence, severity and healing time for recurrent viral infection. Viruses use arginine to replicate.

I use 500 mg L-lysine in vegetarian capsules. I take two to four capsules at a time, once, twice or three times daily. I do this several days a week when I'm feeling well, and every day when I am not. I greatly increase the dose if I have a viral outbreak (usually because I carelessly consumed chocolate, nuts, seeds or glutenous grains). There's no real concern about taking too much. Perhaps the only concern at all would be that you're taking more than you need and wasting money. Amino acids and herbs are generally best taken on an empty stomach (with just water or an herbal tincture like echinacea) for their most potent medicinal effect. Single amino acids and herbs have a "drug-like" (though completely safe) action when they are taken in the right amount, and taken on an empty stomach. Another thing that makes most amino acids and herbs more powerful is taking them on a cyclic schedule (like 3 days on 1 day off for example). Some seem to lose their "punch" if taken in copious quantities every single day.

That said, however, know what each supplement is and does, and take them when you need them!

Melatonin

Melatonin deficiency or "dysfunction in melatonin secretion" is found in migraineurs. This is likely a response to the fact that there is neuronal hyperexcitability. The neuronal hyperexcitability (from either glutamate release or ingestion) of course, leads to an increase in the secretion of CGRP which causes vasodilatation and pain. Remember, there are many "things going on" in a migraine because of the mercury damage to the glutamatergic system.

I take melatonin every night at bedtime (3-5 mg. should suffice, any more is not dangerous, but can cause you to feel extra sleepy the next day). Indeed, studies have shown abnormalities in melatonin secretion in patients who experience migraine and an improvement in migraine following administration of melatonin.

> **Melatonin** levels have been found to be decreased in both migraine and cluster headaches. Melatonin mechanisms are…anti-inflammatory effect, toxic free radical scavenging, reduction of pro-inflammatory cytokine upregulation, **nitric oxide** synthase activity and dopamine release inhibition, membrane stabilisation, GABA and opioid analgesia potentitation, **glutamate neurotoxicity protection**, neurovascular regulation, 5-HT modulation and the similarity in chemical structure to indometacin. [Peres MF et al., Potential therapeutic use of melatonin in migraine and other headache disorders. *Expert Opin Investig Drugs.* 2006 Apr;15(4):367-75.]

Echinacea

I've been taking echinacea for over 20 years. I discovered it when I was in my 30s. I was sick, and was told about a study where blood was taken from an individual and the fighter white blood cells were counted. Then the researchers gave the person echinacea and took the blood again, and the fighter white blood cells had increased many-fold. Echinacea has worked for me for years —

even through all the contradictory reports about whether or not it "worked".

In fact, my children have also taken echinacea all their life. They take echinacea at the first sign of any infection, along with vitamin C, lysine (anti-viral) and colloidal silver (an antimicrobial) and would get well without ever going to a doctor. My children are now 27, 24 and 21, and between the three they've had antibiotics only a few times total. Compare that to a single child usually being given antibiotics sometimes yearly before they're out of elementary school! The benefit of not being given antibiotics is that all three of them have strong immune systems and the proof is that none of them suffers from any chronic illnesses so common today. No asthma, no diabetes, no mental illnesses, no acne, no skin diseases. When they succumb to something like a cold their bodies fight it off as God intended.

I've always known that echinacea worked powerfully, and now I have found that it probably has helped me most all these years because it suppresses excess nitric oxide!

Zhai Z et al. Alcohol extracts of echinacea **inhibit production of nitric oxide** and tumor necrosis factor-alpha by macrophages in vitro. [*Food Agric Immunol.* 2007 Sep;18(3-4):221-236.]

Red Clover Combination

If you have poor elimination, use a supplement called **"Red Clover Combination"** by Nature's Way. It contains a small amount of cascara sagrada, which has been used for centuries to stimulate the intestines, inducing peristalsis, and the elimination of bowel contents. This particular combination does this gently. It is very important to keep the bowels moving and clean. Remember, bad bacteria in the gut will feast upon glucose and create endotoxins that are highly inflammatory, even deadly.

Let's take our cues from Nature once again. A healthy infant eliminates after each meal. As we grow into childhood, we quickly depart from healthy elimination habits because of our highly processed and cooked foods, our busy lives and lack of physical activity. In his book, *Dr. Christopher's Guide to Colon Health* by John R. Christopher, he tells of a gentleman with bowels that contained *years* of fecal buildup – it was 50 pounds or so! He put the man on a few capsules of the herbal combination, starting him slow but building up to taking as many capsules of the combination per day as needed to attain regular and complete evacuations. Once the bowels are clean, the Red Clover Combination can be lowered to where only one capsule daily is needed – sometimes none at all.

Caffeine

Caffeine is actually a natural substance, found in many plants and herbs. It has gotten a "bad rap" because of our overconsumption of coffee at the expense of more healthful beverages, like good, pure water. What you may not know is that caffeine is a powerful vasoconstrictor *because it decreases nitric oxide* [*Pharmacol Res.* 2007 Feb;55(2):96-103.]. It can be good medicine not only as you wean off dangerous drugs, but safely used as a vasocontricting prophylactic against migraines for a lifetime. Properties in coffee that are not healthful have nothing to do with its caffeine content, but with its burnt hydrocarbons, as well as bad fats and sugar put in coffee.

One non-coffee way to make use of caffeine as a vasoconstricting therapy is to use caffeine tablets (found in pharamacies). This way you can take the absolute minimum you need to do the job for you. Purchase 100 mg. tablets and cut them in half. The 50 mg. of caffeine is about what you'd find in a *third* of a cup of coffee. If you can wean down to where you use less and less and are still helped by the caffeine, all the better.

With regard to anyone warning you of a "rebound" effect, consider the alternatives. With or without caffeine, a person with a damaged glutamatergic system will encounter glutamate excesses leading to nitric oxide. The precursors to this are numerous as have been discussed (estrogen drop, alcohol, insulin, glutamate consumption, etc.). Using caffeine in an overall regimen to reduce nitric oxide load is a safe, natural therapy, and far preferable to resorting to dangerous drugs. Anyone who suspects they have a rare allergy to caffeine (I suppose it could happen) shouldn't bother with it, of course. Anyone able to use other methods of keeping nitric oxide levels down *without* using caffeine, should do so, of course.

8 - Get Omega-3 Fatty Acids From Greens

Nearly everyone is *desperately* low in the omega-3 fatty acids. By now most people have heard that omega-3 fatty acids are found in fish. What you may not know is that omega-3 fatty acids are found in fish because fish consume "sea greens", and it is from the sea greens they get the building blocks of the fatty acid. The other thing most people still don't know is that omega-3 fatty acids are instantly destroyed by heat, air, and light. So any amount of cooking fish would turn a highly beneficial fat into a highly damaging fat, anyway, and here is why:

The **omega-3 fatty acid** is an 18 carbon chain molecule with *three* sites on the molecule that are "double bonds". These are sites where Nature designed that the molecule be "electric" and able to interact with your cells in a healthful way.

Omega-3 FATTY ACID
C=Carbon H=Hydrogen
Note the "double bond" at the 3rd, 6th and 9th Carbon.
The Carbon atom has four electron sites surrounding it that wants to be paired – hence the need for four bonds around each Carbon
Also note the missing Hydrogens at the double bonds – these are places on the molecule that are "electric" and where the molecule can react or attach to needed areas/cells in the body.
The Carbon attached to an "OH" group with a double bond to an Oxygen is called a Carboxyl group on the end of the fatty acid. Carboxyl groups are present in all fatty acids.
B. Tancredi BSc, CN

Note in the above drawing that there are 18 "C"s – these are carbons, the basis of an organic molecule. Note that if you count over from the first carbon on the left (follow the curve), on the third carbon is the first double bond. This is how omega-3 fatty acids are named, i.e., three omega (three from the end). **Omega-6 fatty acids** (found mostly in vegetable oils, nuts and seeds) have only two double bonds in their unoxidized, unhydrogenated (natural) state. The first double bond starts on the sixth carbon (there would be no double bond on the third carbon). Omega-6 is also a "bent" molecule, but less so than the omega-3. Double bonds are "tension" sites, making the molecule bent, unstable, reactive, and "electric".

Molecules with double bonds are molecules on a mission (looking to accept another atom at the double bond site, which breaks the double bond (it becomes a single bond) and the molecule becomes "stable"). This is how an *unoxidized* fatty acid molecule (oxidation occurs when the double bond is broken by an oxygen atom) can incorporate into your cell membranes. That double bond is necessary for the molecule to do its beneficial work.

Omega-9 fatty acids have only one double bond, on the ninth carbon. These molecules are the least bent of the "unsaturated" fatty acids. Omega-9 fatty acids are found primarily in olive and avocado oils. They are less bent, so the molecules can stack on top of each other. This is why olive oil "hardens" when you refrigerate it. Omega-9 fatty acids are mono-unsaturated. Omega-3 and omega-6 fatty acids are poly-unsaturated. Mono = one site of unsaturation; poly = more than one site of unsaturation (unsaturatation means a double bond).

Its not that omega-9 fats are *better* for you, it is that they are far less damaging when oxidized than an omega-3 by virtue of only one site that is oxidized, compared to three sites of potential oxidation. However, extra virgin olive oil is perhaps the very best mono-unsaturated oil because it has many powerful antioxidants in it as well (phytochemicals).

The study below is saying that omega-9 fatty acids are *non-essential* and actually interfere with the healthful anti-inflammatory process of the *essential* fatty acids in the omega-3 family. From omega-3 fatty acids, the body can make all the omega-6 and omega-9 it needs. So omega-3 is very important to consume in the diet every day. But they *must* be completely unoxidized to be of benefit and to also not be harmful (oxidized fatty acids are "free radicals" and cause great harm in the body).

...theories of atherosclerosis (my note: which is caused by **inflammation** within arteries) may have considerably exaggerated the importance of **oxidized lipoprotein** and vascular inflammation ...one new and basic question is whether the biology of essential dietary lipids may help us understand the role of the inflammatory process ...**omega-3** [a] precursor of major mediators of inflammation .... on the other hand **non-essential lipids** (**omega-9** and saturated fatty acids) interfere with biological activities of essential lipids. [*Subcell Biochem* 2007;42:283-97.]

The double bonds of all three of the aforementioned unsaturated fats are easily broken by heat, air or light. It is wisest to treat all unsaturated fatty acids with the gentlest of care so that you can consume the molecule in the most healthful state possible, or it would be better to consume no fats at all. The truth is, fats are healthful in their unoxidized natural state, and disease-promoting in their hydrogenated, oxidized or altered state.

One example of an altered fat is a **"trans" fat**. This is where man has so altered the fatty acid molecule that it is stable to the point of ridiculousness. In our desire for "shelf life" of food with fats (to not have fats oxidize which is what turning *rancid* is) man has created a monster. Trans fats are "backwards" fats the body not only does not recognize, but they are now fats that "attack" the body's cells, causing great damage. Trans fats are worse than hydrogenated fats.

So what are **hydrogenated fats**? If the double bond site gets "filled" by a hydrogen atom, the fat molecule becomes *hydrogenated*. You've heard how "hydrogenated" fats aren't healthful. In an omega-3 fatty acid, the molecules are so bent, they cannot stack tightly together. This makes them liquid, as well as very reactive in the body, *and* easily oxidizable (and thus easily spoiled, i.e., *rancid*). This very liquid fat doesn't harden when put in the refrigerator – *and it also doesn't harden when put into your body*. That's a good thing. Omega-3 fatty acids create healthful "fluid" membranes around your cells, and "fluid" blood that doesn't abnormally clump or clot. But when you break the double bond sites by inserting hydrogen atoms, the molecule becomes "stable", it straightens out, and the molecules can now stack tightly upon each other. Because they can "stack", they harden, are no longer liquid, but also cannot create fluid cell membranes or blood.

Hydrogenating is how food manufacturers take a liquid oil and create a hard oil (for example changing oil into margarine). Hydrogenated fats aren't so harmful as they are perfectly useless. Hydrogenated fats are also called "saturated" fats, and are actually found in Nature. Coconut oil is a good example. There's nothing terribly wrong with consuming coconut oil. The harm of saturated fats comes when they become the main source of fats in the body, at the expense of healthful fatty acids the body needs to make healthy cells. From unsaturated fatty acids, your body can actually make all the "saturated fats" it needs (and it *does* need a certain amount). To summarize, hydrogenated or saturated fats have no double bonds with which to interact with your cell's membranes and thus participate in many healthful reactions. *Partially hydrogenated* fats are far worse than hydrogenated in that they partially interact, and thus can and do get in the way of the beneficial fats doing their good work.

Among the worst fats are **"oxidized" fats.** Oxidized fats are *any* fat that once had a double bond, now has an oxygen atom attached to the molecule where the double bond once was, turning it from a good fat into a "free radical". The double bond is broken and the open site is filled with an oxygen atom. The problem is that an oxygen atom has an electron floating around in its outer orbit looking for a "mate". It will steal from other atoms to get that mate, *damaging the other molecule* of which that atom is a part. This is what it means when you hear "free radical" damage. What is free radical damage? The best analogy I've ever heard is that of a metal picnic table. A new metal picnic table with its fresh coat of paint can endure rain and sunhine for perhaps a year or two. But then as the paint wears off and the metal underneath is exposed, the oxygen in the air will begin to react with the metal. This is a "free radical" reaction, and it causes *rust.* When free radicals are continually created or introduced into your body, the damage done to your 10-100 trillion cells is like a "rusting" of sorts. The extra electron on the oxygen steals from other atoms, doing damage throughout the entire body. Ultimately, this leads to all manner of disease and pain if not stopped. How do you stop it? *Antioxidants!*

The Importance Of Unoxidized Omega-3 Fatty Acids

How much unoxidized omega-3 does your body need? The only thing science has *proven* is that you need more omega-3 than omega-6, and in fact, an excess of omega-6 will keep omega-3 from doing the good job it is supposed to do. Again, if you *only* consumed omega-3 (not possible, but let's assume) you'd be way ahead of the game because from it your body can make all the other fats it wants/needs.

I found one study claiming that oxidized omega-3 worked better than unoxidized as an antiinflammatory [Mishra et al 2004] The truth is, we know that oxidation creates an oxygen "free radical" which attacks cells. In this study, did the oxygen free radical stimulate an "antioxidant response"? That's one way alcohol is of benefit (by attacking your cells) and is why you're told to consume no more than about 4 ounces a day. But deliberately attacking your cells and hoping for a protective response wouldn't work in people with damaged protective mechanisms. Stick to God's wisdom, and consume all fats as unaltered and unoxidized as possible. If your body needs anything oxidized, it will do it for you!

So all fats should be consumed unoxidized (and unhydrogenated). But in cases where the body is chronically ill, this isn't merely an option, it is mandatory for healing. Therefore, use only organic extra virgin olive oil in dressing salads and only put it on food *after* cooking. Unfortunately, due to our polluted waters I strongly believe it is no longer safe to consume fish or their oils (even krill) or any blue-green algaes or other sea greens (these have a high affinity for mercury outside of the body as well). A study found at pubmed.gov states that Krill oil (which *may* rightfully claim to have no mercury — I don't know) but it is actually high in cadmium!

The results show relatively **high levels of cadmium in krill**, which is assumed to be the main reason for the high levels of cadmium in petrels and skuas. [Nygård T, et al. Metal dynamics in an Antarctic food chain. *Mar Pollut Bull.* 2001 Jul;42(7):598-602]

At www.medfinds.com the alarm is sounded as well warning that blue-green algae can accumulate heavy metals from contaminated water. They say that consuming blue-green algae could, in theory, increase the body's load of lead, mercury, and cadmium. For those who are <u>not</u> sick or suffering, this threat likely doesn't seem real at all. The health store shelves are full of these types of supplements. But when you're already damaged by mercury and suffering, you need to do everything humanly possible to not ingest *any* more toxic metals. In addition, medfinds says that samples of spirulina (a type of blue-green algae) have also been found to be contaminated with animal hairs and insect fragments. Another popular species of blue-green algae, *Aphanizomenon flos-aquae*, has been found to produce toxins. Until I can be convinced otherwise, anything from our polluted waters is to be avoided.

Avoid butter (a saturated fat) except small amounts of organic, raw butter (do not cook with it).

Looking at the subject of omega-3 fatty acids from God or Nature's point of view, it makes no sense that a person with a damaged glutamatergic system, and especially with fluctuating hormones such as those that cause a monthly migraine, use any concentrated form of omega-3 oils in an attempt to get their omega-3 fatty acids. The problem is that the concentrated omega-3 could artificially alter hormone levels to an unnatural "high", causing a resultant plummet and worsening symptoms, especially migraines.

Indeed, if flax were supposed to be a source of omega-3 fatty acids in human nutrition, we would be able to extract it from the whole seed by mere chewing. Anyone who has eaten a whole flax seed knows this just doesn't happen (flax exits the body pretty much the way it entered it). Instead, manufacturers use state-of-the-art methods to carefully extract the oil from the tiny seed and also must take great pains to not oxidize the fatty acids. The oil is kept refrigerated and in dark brown or black bottles. With all that in mind, consider this: *Where does a cow get omega-3?*

The answer, is from grass. Likewise, you are supposed to obtain all the essential fatty acids you need when you consume a diet of mostly raw vegetables and fruits with lots of raw greens. This is especially true as long as you also no longer consume oxidized fats, trans fats, hydrogenated and partially hydrogenated fats, etc. Now consider yet another thing: How many people do you know still alive in their 80's or 90's and yet they never took any fish or flax oil supplements?

There's also a lot of research that has been done into omega-3 and omega-6 (the essential fatty acids that we all need to be healthy) and all of the evidence that we have come across definitely indicates that grass fed beef (and the eggs that come from our grass fed chickens) have a much, much better ratio of omega-3 to omega-6 than grain fed animals. "Diet can significantly alter the fatty acid composition in fed cattle. Cattle fed primarily **grass enhanced the omega-3 content of beef by 60%** and also produces a more favorable omega-6 to omega-3 ratio. Conventional [grain fed] beef contains a 4:1 6:3 ratio while grass only diets produce a 2:1 6:3 ratio". [www.csuchico.edu/agr/grsfdbef/health-benefits/ben-03-06.html]

This doesn't mean you are supposed to get the omega-3 fatty acids "secondhand" by eating the beef. Cooking beef would oxidize the omega-3 fatty acids (as it does when you cook fish). This *does* mean that you, too, can consume copious quantities of greens every day for enhancing the omega-3 fatty acid content of your body (not to mention the other fabulous benefits derived from greens).

<u>What About Cholesterol?</u>

The issue of cholesterol, and the fact that there is a hidden real truth, can be applied to all of nutrition. For many years the recommendation was to be on a low fat, low cholesterol diet. Why? Because plaques in arteries were found to be made up of cholesterol. The fact that they are also made up of calcium doesn't get the same "press". Indeed, there are two truths that you've likely never been told, and actually, few understand. The ones who understand the *least* seem to be doctors, only as proven by the thousands upon thousands of cholesterol-lowering drugs still being prescribed. Indeed, artificially lowering your cholesterol is extremely dangerous and has now been linked with neurological disorders, like Parkinson's. In fact, the advertising by-line that says something about a "rare" side-effect of taking cholesterol-lowering drugs is muscle weakness, is an outright lie. Just go on "Lipitor" (cholesterol lowering drug) blog sites and you will find thousands of people complaining about muscle weakness and various illnesses they suspect are from the Lipitor.

The two facts not shared with you are that cholesterol is *not* the culprit in cardiovascular disease, atherosclerosis, arteriosclerosis, etc. The real culprit is inflammation and resultant damage to the lining of your arteries. Cholesterol can contribute to the inflammation when it is *oxidized* but it also participates in the attempt to heal damaged arteries by joinging with calcium to "patch up" (harden) a damaged area. If your artery was damaged so badly that an actual hole was created, you could bleed to death. Unfortunately, when the underlying cause of the damage (inflammation caused by oxygen free radicals, various chemicals, and lack of various protective antioxidants) is never addressed, the damage continues, and so does the "repair" (hardening).

So here is the second thing you're not told, and it's huge: There is absolutely nothing wrong with cholesterol. In fact, cholesterol is the precursor to many hormones and is absolutely essential. Artificial attempts to lower it take away the building blocks for hormones and can cause all manner of misery and illness. Cholesterol is the fat molecule that lines your arteries making them slick as glass so your blood can rush around your body at break-neck speed. That cholesterol lining provides the protective surface needed to prevent excessive friction from the rushing blood. Cholesterol is a 27-carbon chain fat, and in its natural state has multiple sites of "double bonds", meaning sites where it has "electric" potential, or the ability to interact with your cells and do the things its suppose to do. If those "double bonds" are broken by hydrogen or oxygen, the molecule becomes "saturated", hardened, or a "free radical".

The truth is, oxidized cholesterol behaves as an *oxidant* (a free radical, damaging your cells and arteries), and unoxidized cholesterol behaves as an antioxidant (healing, protective). High HDL has always been considered protective while high LDL has always been considered a high risk marker for cardiovascular disease. It appears that HDL's intended job is to carry *good* (unoxidized) cholesterol for use and/or disposal (as needed) while LDL carries *oxidized* cholesterol around the body, depositing it where it does harm. The "functional properties" spoken of in the text box below could very well mean that the body needs to produce healthy "high density lipoprotein" as well as produce or consume unoxidized cholesterol. It is *oxidized* cholesterol that is found in hardened arteries. Indeed, unheated cholesterol sources (like raw butter, and raw eggs) is why some "health foodists" put raw eggs into their smoothies, and use raw butter. On a personal note, my husband and I use raw butter and raw egg yolks whenever we want, and blood tests show that our cholesterol levels haven't gone up one iota because of it.

Although a low level of high-density lipoprotein **(HDL) cholesterol** is a useful clinical predictor of coronary heart disease, raising the HDL cholesterol level does not necessarily lower this risk. Part of the explanation for this paradox may be that, under certain conditions, HDL either can be less functional as an antioxidant or can even enhance the oxidation and inflammation associated with atherosclerotic plaque. Thus, the functional properties of HDL—not simply the level—may need to be considered and optimized. [Ansell BJ. The two faces of the 'good' cholesterol. *Cleve Clin J Med* 2007 Oct;74(10):697-700, 703-5.]

In fact, the best oils are found in whole, raw nuts, seeds and avocadoes (although nuts and seeds should be avoided by people with viral problems or cancer). But you can also use organic, extra virgin olive oil, especially unheated on salads, or put on foods after cooking. Those "amber" color oils (highly processed), sold in clear bottles where the light can damage the fat molecules even more are to be shunned forevermore.

Relatively large quantities of hydroperoxides (Ch18:2-00H) and some hydroxides of Ch18:2 (Ch18:2-OH) are formed during the early stages of in vitro **peroxidation of LDL and HDL**, and these two forms of oxidized Ch18:2 are **present in human atherosclerotic lesions**. [Julie K. Christhon et al. *Journal of Lipid Research* Volume 36, 1995]

---

9 - Supplements For Protecting Your Liver and Kidneys, And For "Detox"

Milk Thistle

The active components in milk thistle are powerful protectors of the liver. In fact turmeric and milk thistle are often recommended together for general liver health as well as powerful antidotes to toxic substances suffered by the liver. For example, laboratory mice were given poisonous mushrooms. One group was also given "silybin" an active component in milk thistle. The group that received the silybin lived. The group that did not receive the silybin died.

> At present, the most effective clinical antidote to acute Amanita phalloides **mushroom poisoning** is **silybin**, an antioxidant possessing free radical scavenger activity and inhibiting lipid peroxidation, stabilizing membrane structure and protecting enzymes under conditions of oxidative stress. [*Med Hypotheses* 2007;69(2):361-7.]

Vitamin C

Of the thousands of antioxidant compounds found in Nature, most people only know of vitamin C. "Antioxidant" means that it disables or eliminates oxygen free radicals. But what most people don't know is that the toxicity of substances has to do with the substance's ability to attack your cells as a "free radical". I had an amazing detox experience with vitamin C recently (as I also shared in Chapter 3).

Every morning I take all of my "morning" supplements, which includes 500 mg. of vitamin C. One particular morning I had a dental appointment which was to include conscious sedation and I was told to not take any food or anything. So of course I did not take my supplements. I took the sedation pill, and within 15 minutes was *out.* Then, a few weeks later I didn't know I would be having conscious sedation, so I had taken my supplements, including the "C". *The sedation pill took over 2 hours to work, and then wore off quickly!*

I've had subsequent experiences on mornings where I'd taken the vitamin "C", then shots of anesthesia wouldn't work, and the dentist would keep giving additional shots until he was afraid to give any more. On the days I didn't take vitamin C I didn't have that problem at all. This has shown me firsthand how vitamin C is a powerful detoxifier! The recommendation is to take vitamin C *after* any encounter with medical toxins, including anesthesia.

10 - Supplements & Therapies Specifically For Multiple Sclerosis

All of the above supplements are for MS which has viral, glutamatergic damage, and inflammation as part all the things going on. But the one supplement that is truly a miracle for MS symptoms is Ca-AEP. Ca-AEP, taken along with stopping further mercury damage, and addressing inflammation with antiinflammatory diet and supplements is about the best you can do apart from getting stem cells some day.

Ca-AEP

Calcium 2-AEP (Calcium 2-Aminoethanol Phosphate) or CaAEP for short, is a vitamin-like metabolite and a crucial part of your cell membrane's integrity. It acts to bind fatty acids of the cell membrane structure, carry electrolytes and essential nutrients into cells, protect the cell from harmful agents, repairs cell neurotransmission and binds minerals to cell membranes to serve as electrical condensers. Nutritionally-oriented doctors may use it for sclerotic disorders (like multiple sclerosis, atherosclerosis, and systemic sclerosis) inflammatory disorders, diabetes and its complications, osteoporosis, lung diseases and immune disorders.

CaAEP has been found to be a potent sensitizer of hypothalamic function (a part of the brain). *Without CaAEP there would be a loss of cellular electrical charge.* CaAEP is a necessary component of cell membrane integrity and cell sensitivity, and is missing when damage to neurons and damage to the myelin sheath occur as in multiple sclerosis. CaAEP binds fatty acids and electrolytes to the cell membrane structure that generates the cell's ability to connect with other cells. There have been many studies done over the course of 30 years that have proven CaAEP's benefit for neurotransmission, nerve impulse generation and muscular contractions. Most of the work with CaAEP was done by Hans A. Nieper, M.D. of Hannover, Germany.

I was talking to a young man with MS once and I asked him how much CaAEP he was taking. He said, "I used to take that. It doesn't work for me anymore". This young man illustrates the problem with drugs vs. supplements. People take a tiny prescription pill once a day for something, so when it comes to taking supplements they think the dose should be the same — one tiny pill. But supplements are more like food than drugs — although *powerful* and with miraculous compounds God put there for the body's healing. In the case of CaAEP, while the bottle may say take 2 per day in divided doses — that's the "FDA" label. The FDA label is the one written so as not to attract the scrutiny and ire of the FDA who likes to tell supplement manufacturers what they can and cannot say. However, studies that are conducted, proving the efficacy of a supplement nearly always safely use many times more than what the bottle is allowed to say. That young man *may* have continued to reap benefit from the CaAEP, had he increased the dose as needed.

Know why you are taking each and every supplement, and purchase only from reputable manufacturers. Only in this way can you hope to take the right amount for you. I prefer the quality and reputation of the Ca-AEP made by Vitamin Research Products, available at www.vrp.com.

2,000 patients were treated in Germany over 24 years revealing greater efficacy from **Ca-AEP** treatments than other known treatment. In 1986, Dr. George Morrissette conducted a retrospective poll of patients in the USA who originally had begun Ca-AEP treatment in Germany for MS. 82% of the almost 300 patients that entered the study showed a positive benefit from Ca-AEP therapy. And when treatment began in the early stages of MS, positive results rose to 92%. Long-term observation of Ca-AEP's effects on more than 2,000 MS patients revealed a host of additional benefits. MS patients receiving Ca-AEP showed less signs of aging in their outward appearance, increased tissue elasticity and skeletal firmness and a marked absence of osteoporosis. Second to the destruction of the myelin sheath of the nerve fibers, MS patients are especially at risk of kidney infection due to insufficient membrane polarization at the cellular level. The supplementation of Ca-AEP repairs cell membrane function and maintains it at optimal levels. It raises the depressed energy in the membrane system of the nerves' myelin sheath of MS patients by several-fold, restoring proper synaptic function in the affected organs. Treatment with Ca-AEP is non-toxic. [by Ward Dean, MD and Jim English. http://www.nutrition-review.org/library/calcium_aep.html]

Lipoic Acid

Lipoic acid functions as a potent antioxidant by helping protect cells from the damaging effects of free radicals. Besides protecting membranes, mitochondria (the energy-producing structures within cells) and cellular DNA, lipoic acid works synergistically with vitamins C and E and CoQ10 — all also antioxidants. Note in the study below how patients safely took 1,200 mg. of lipoic acid twice daily. Most lipoic acid supplements are 100 or 300 mg. So you see that you could take several of the 100 mg. or a couple of the 300 mg. three or four times a day with great benefit, and no danger whatsoever. Again, the problem with people thinking supplements don't work, is often that they don't take enough — or they don't stop polluting their body first but expect supplements to "bail them out" of their erroneous ways.

When you take lipoic acid you will notice a "sulfur" smell when you urinate. This is normal. Sulfur is a central component of many natural compounds that make up proteins and chelate [remove] heavy metals from the body.

> 37 patients were randomly assigned to one of four groups that received: 1) placebo twice daily; 2) 600 mg of **lipoic acid** twice daily; 3) 1200 mg of lipoic acid in the morning and placebo in the evening; and 4) 1200 mg of lipoic acid twice daily. Lipoic acid **decreased the two inflammatory mediators** in a dose-dependent fashion. In animal studies, such changes have been associated with **decreased progression of multiple sclerosis.** None of these doses proved toxic. [Yadav V et al. Lipoic acid in multiple sclerosis: a pilot study. *Mult Scler* 2005 Apr;11(2):159-65.]

Lipoic acid has been shown to "spare" glutathione – meaning it helps your body produce and keep more glutathione. (Refer to Chapter 7 *Psoriasis*). In fact, perhaps the best reason to take lipoic acid is for its glutathione-sparing activity. Alpha lipoic has to be converted to R-lipoic acid in the body, so many people take the more expensive R-lipoic acid. Recall that glutathione is one of the most important detoxifiers we know of in the body. If you go to a hospital with an acetaminophen overdose, for example, you'll be given an intravenous supplement to boost glutathione as a detoxifier of the poison.

> When seven healthy people were given a single application of up to 3,000 mg of glutathione, there was **no** increase in blood glutathione levels. The human gastrointestinal tract contains significant amounts of an enzyme (gamma-glutamyltranspeptidase) that breaks down glutathione. [Witschi A, Reddy S, Stofer B, Lauterburg BH. The systemic availability of oral glutathione. *Eur J Clin Pharmacol* 1992;43:667-9.]

The study clearly shows that giving glutathione as a supplement is *not* the best way to obtain it. In fact, people whose bodies and brains have been damaged by mercury will likely have a terrible reaction to preformed glutathione (e.g., as a supplement or an I.V.). This is because glutathione is a "tripeptide", made up of the three amino acids glutamine (the precursor to glutamate), cysteine and glycine. If you have a damaged glutamatergic system, taking glutamine can end painfully – like with a three day migraine.

Instead, researchers have found that supplying the body with all it needs nutritionally is the best way to increase your glutathione levels. The best way to do this are vitamin C, lipoic acid, plant foods rich in sulfur like broccoli, brussels sprouts or cabbage, a B-complex supplement and selenium (found in garlic, mushrooms and asparagus). All of these are required in the manufacture of glutathione, along with several amino acids you will get by consuming a diet of whole plants foods.

…in one trial, blood glutathione levels rose nearly 50% in healthy people taking **500 mg of vitamin C** per day for only two weeks. [Johnston CS, Meyer CG, Srilakshmi JC. Vitamin C **elevates red blood cell glutathione** in healthy adults. *Am J Clin Nutr* 1993;58:103-5.]

Dietary sulfur amino acid content is a major determinant of glutathione concentration in some tissues. [**Sulfur amino acid deficiency depresses brain glutathione concentration** *Nutr Neurosci* 2001;4(3):213-22]

Ginkgo

The antioxidant compounds in ginkgo have an affinity for the brain. In numerous studies these compounds have been found to protect neurons from oxidative damage and death.

These results suggest that the **neuroprotective effects of ginkgo biloba** extract are partly associated with its antioxidant properties and highlight its possible effectiveness in neurodegenerative diseases (such as Alzheimer's) via the inhibition of Abeta-induced toxicity and cell death. [S. Bastianetto et al. The ginkgo biloba extract (Egb 761) protects hippocampal neurons against cell death induced by beta amyloid. Eur J Neurosci (2000) 12: 1882-90]

L-Lysine

Part of the misery suffered in MS, migraines and bodies damaged by mercury in general, is the agony of viral outbreaks. These outbreaks are not only painful, but cause damage to cells, further exacerbating symptoms associated with the disease. What is not understood, even by many in the medical community, is that an outbreak is actually more often *not visible* than visible. I went to a doctor for trigeminal pain and when I suggested that it was from herpes, I was all but laughed at. I insisted on a blood test. Grudgingly, the doctor ordered a herpes simplex virus (HSV) type 1 and type 2 test for antibodies IgG and IgM. IgG and IgM are antibodies the body produces in response to an infection. Antibodies are what work to prevent infectious agents from being able to infect.

If the results for the IgG came back .89 or less then I would be "negative" for detectable HSV 1 or 2. If the results came back .90-1.09 the results would mean "equivocal" and the doctor might do a repeat test in a week or two. If the results came back 1.10 or higher, then I would be "positive" for current but also past HSV 1 or 2 infection.

Then for the IgM test, if the results came back .89 or less I would be "negative" for HSV IgM antibody. If .90-1.09 the test would be considered "equivocal" and a repeat test might be ordered. If the results were 1.10 or higher, I would be considered "positive" for IgM antibody to HSV 1 and/or 2 which would mean that I had an infection and it is likely more current. So the higher either of these, the greater the infection.

My results: IgG <u>39.8</u> and IgM <u>1.76</u>.

The doctor called and left the results on my answering machine. This was a few days after I'd gone to that doctor with the horrific pain of trigeminal neuralgia. While awaiting the test results, I had already begun anti-viral therapies on my own because I was certain I had a major herpes outbreak (or we'll coin a new term and call it an "inbreak"). Within 24-hours I had it under control. The phone call confirmed my own diagnosis.

The first therapy for a herpes outbreak or inbreak is L-lysine, mentioned in the nitric oxide squelchers section. I have found the following statement to be completely true in my own battle against herpes outbreaks:

L-lysine is an amino acid that is essential building block for proteins. L-lysine has been proven as effective as prescription drugs in fighting herpes. 2000 mg. daily [http://www.hsv-free.com/Herpes_cure_info.htm]

When I know I'm having an outbreak or inbreak of herpes (can be anything from pain or fullness in ears, fluctuating eyesight, sore throats, extreme tiredness, hip pain or more) I'll take four 500 mg. vege caps of L-lysine *every 4 hours* while awake until the symptoms subside. I usually use "Insure Herbal" (a mixture of echinacea and goldenseal) in water as the liquid used to take the pills. Then between outbreaks and inbreaks I take two 500 mg. vege caps of L-lysine every few days. I always follow a low arginine diet.

Electricity Kills Pathogens: The Zapper

Parasites (that means viruses, bacteria, fungi and worms) cannot defend their positive polarity (shortage of electrons) against the introduction of simple direct current and they die very quickly. Negative ions will repel parasites whether electric current, magnets, or orgone generates the ions. **Parasites** not only **die when subjected to electricity**, but also disintegrate and are easily assimilated as harmless nutrients or eliminated. [Don Croft, the developer and manufacturer of the Terminator II Zapper.]

I have several zappers. Below are recommended websites where you can see the zappers and read in detail about how and why they work. I have several styles because getting pathogens "zapped" is so important to healing and well-being, that I use them all, but at different times to make sure the job is getting done. I am certain, however, that you only *need* one good zapper. One zapper has copper handholds which I can lay and watch TV and use (either 7 minutes on, 20 minute off cycle Dr. Hulda Clark recommends in "The Cure For All Cancers" or for a continuous 60 minutes others recommend). For hands-free, I put the copper electrodes under my arms while I'm working on the computer. One electrode is attached to a green wire, and one is attached to a red wire. I alternate the red wire to the right side one zapping, and then to the left side the next zapping. Apparently, the red side will be the side that packs the most punch to the parasites.

Another zapper I have has copper plates that can be put on the floor and you place your feet on them for zapping. I haven't found this to be terribly convenient, as I rarely sit still, much less with my feet squarely on the floor. The wristbands are not considered the most effective way to zap, so I don't use them. I have a "Terminator" zapper that has two copper circles as the electrodes. You place the entire little unit against your body to zap. I use this for a few hours at night. With any zapper, you have to educate yourself to be motivated and to use it properly. No-one has ever been electrocuted (it's a 9 volt battery!) nor harmed from a zapper. You'd have to be persistent and do something quite dramatic, like trying to alter the electronics or try to plug the unit into a wall outlet or something, to do any harm to yourself. The websites explain where, when and who should and should not use a zapper.

So again, the best recommendation is to do your own homework and decide which style of zapper is most compatible with your lifestyle. Go to www.toolsforhealing.com or www.paradevices.com. If the concept of "electrocuting" parasites is new to you, you need to know that it is actually not at all new, and is based on science. What the doctors below found applies to an electrical current being applied directly to a virus. Unfortunately, viruses hide within cells and cannot be so easily killed. This is where the "Rife" machines enter (see below).

...a great step was taken in the war against viruses and bacteria when doctors William Lyman and Steven Kaali made an astonishing announcement on March 14th of 1991 at the First International Symposium on Combination Therapies. Lyman and Kaali, researchers from the Albert Einstein School of Medicine, reported that a small amount of electric current, flowing through a dish of fluid containing the HIV virus, reduced its ability to infect cells by up to 95%! The electric current used was very small, (only 50-100 microamperes) which is safe for blood cells but harmful to viruses and other pathogens. The announcement was reported in Science News, Longevity Magazine, and the Houston Post. Unfortunately, further media coverage of this breakthrough was suppressed. [Mike Forrest Feb 6, 1998]

Frequencies Kill Pathogens: The Rife Machine

Another way to "zap" pathogens is with sound frequencies. In the early 1900's Doctor Raymond Royal Rife (born in 1888) discovered that all organisms, viruses, bacteria molds, and fungus, vibrate at a specific frequency. The results are similar as obtained with the electric pulse frequency of zapping. Dr. Rife observed that *if bombarded by the same frequency, at which it vibrated, a particular pathogen would explode and be destroyed.* There are actually photos taken under the microscope that show this to be true.

Furthermore, unlike organisms treated with antibiotics (e.g., staphylococcus, streptococcus, chicken pox virus, etc.) those that were treated with the matching frequencies did not go on to form new strains resistant to antibiotics.

Doctor Rife's original research was substantiated to be one of the most effective approaches to treat all diseases. Fortunately, there has been a new interest in Rife's technology and diseases like shingles have been shown to be eradicated! Read all about Dr. Rife at www.wikipedia.com. He claimed to cure cancer, and then claimed that the American Medical Association had sabotaged his work. Knowing what I've witnessed firsthand with doctors being sabotaged by agencies who have their own "special interests" (which really means how much money they'd lose if healthcare professionals or "regular" people were able to cure their diseases completely and inexpensively), I'd have to say that I believe Dr. Rife's claim. See: http://www.rife-machine.com/index.htm.

Dr. Royal R. Rife believed that the frequencies generated by a frequency/function generator would enter the body and devitalize targeted organisms. In other words, he discovered that all viruses, bacteria, parasites and other pathogens are particularly sensitive to a specific resonant "frequency" of sound and can be destroyed by intensifying that frequency until they literally explode like an intense musical note that can shatter a wine glass! [http://newhopetechnologies.com/electromedicine.htm]

Unfortunately a Rife machine is expensive (in the thousands). I think it would be well worth the investment, however. If you were to only purchase one machine, and you can afford the Rife machine, you might want to consider that it be the one you purchase. This means you must make sure you are purchasing a machine based on Rife's work. When I began my investigations, I found "Rife" machines that were really just "glorified zappers". In fact, when I asked one seller of a machine they called a Rife machine, he told me point blank that his machine was a "better" zapper. He said it could generate more electricity. As I was talking to him I was using my own zapper at 2500 hertz. That generates quite a "tingle", and I couldn't imagine tolerating any more. I asked if more hertz would hurt, and he agreed that it could. It became clear that this was *not* a true Rife machine – it was electricity pure and simple, and not sound waves.

After much searching, I found several websites that *appear* to be using true Rife technology. Then I found Ron Strauss, *Educator and Consultant in electromagnetic healing and Rife technology.* Ron shared with me at length various facts about electromagnetic healing and so much more. Ron can be reached at rstrauss@mchsi.com. Ron and I discussed how there is so much more to know than any one human being will ever know, but if we each adhere to basic truths we will be doing the very best we can do for genuine healing.

Indeed, the key to success with these therapies (zapping or Rife) would be that they are used in combination with the best possible diet (described below), and that they are indeed *used*, not abandoned. You can't use them once and think you should be cured forever. In fact, the most common complaints I hear from people who are very ill is "how many" supplements they should be taking, or how "difficult" it is to change their diet. Every human being wants convenience and to not have their life disrupted by things they *must* do instead of things they want to do. True healing can only come about and be maintained on a program that is followed daily for the rest of a person's life.

Ozonated Water

Dr. R. Mattassi at the Santa Corona Hospital in Milan, Italy treated 27 herpes patients with increased oxygenation. These patients received from only one to a maximum of five injections of oxygen (O2 and O3). All 27 patients were declared completely healed. Five years later, with no further treatment, 24 of the 27 were still outbreak and symptom free. Re-infection was suspected in the other three. Unbelievably, in the United States, using "ozone" therapies is illegal. Many doctors know about ozone and some have even secretly used it. Some non-medical practitioners still use it under their rights to use any "natural" therapies as they deem safe and effective.

Viruses are anaerobic, and thus are killed by oxygen. This is why a healthy, oxygenated body is the goal for everyone, but is *especially* important for people with dormant herpes. Recall that over 85% of all people have or will get some form of herpes. Increasing oxygenation at the cellular level has been proven to be done by oral ingestion of O2 or O3, such as the use of ozonated water or hydrogen peroxide. There are other oxygenation therapies, such as rectal insufflations of ozone, intravenous injections of oxygen, hydrogen peroxide or hyperbaric chambers. Some are expensive, some are painful, and some aren't allowed in the United States. I choose to ozonate the air of my home, and to ozonate the water I drink.

One water ozonator is the "Nature-Kleen" ozonator. An excellent source for this is www.toolsforwellness.com. The website explains how to use the machine.

Ali Demirci, an associate professor of agricultural and biological engineering at Pennsylvania State University, investigating the use of ozone: **Ozone** has been proven to be a more effective antimicrobial than the most commonly used disinfectant, chlorine, against a wide range of micro-organisms." *Ozone has certain characteristics that make it attractive for use as a sanitizer in food processing,"* Demirci stated. *"It is a strong antimicrobial agent with high reactivity and spontaneous decomposition to a non-toxic product — oxygen."* [Scientists explore pathogen killing methods without heat. Ahmed ElAmin, April 3, 2006.]

11 - Pure, Whole, Fresh, Preferably Organic, Plant-Food Diet

Plant polyphenols, a large group of natural antioxidants, are serious candidates in explanations of the protective effects of vegetables and fruits against cancer and cardiovascular diseases. ... vegetables and fruits contain compounds that have protective effects, independent of those of known nutrients and micronutrients.... **over 6,000 different flavonoids occurring in plants have been described**...polyphenols...trap and scavenge free radicals, regulate nitric oxide, decrease leukocyte immobilization, induce apoptosis, inhibit cell proliferation and angiogenesis, and exhibit phytoestrogenic activity...bacteria present in the human colon metabolize polyphenols....[Ilja CW Arts and Peter CH Hollman. Polyphenols and disease risk in epidemiologic studies. *American Journal of Clinical Nutrition.*Vol. 81, No. 1, 317S-325S, January 2005]

You need to seek out organic foods because they are grown without pesticides and other dangerous chemicals. I cannot believe how many people think that "organic" means "health food" and bad taste. If you ask most people what "organic" means, they are clueless, both as to the definition of organically-grown, and as to the importance. "Certified Organic" has the government stamp of approval, and growers must prove that the ground upon which the produce is grown is free of pesticides. There are stringent guidelines these growers must prove and maintain.

There are not many studies proving that organic produce is superior (there is little financial incentive to do these types of studies), but those of us that buy organic *know* the nutrients are higher. However, there is one study that shows a much higher level of various antioxidants in organically-grown tomatoes over commerically grown. I feel certain that if someone were to do a similar study on all other organic vs. commerically-grown produce, the results would be the same - *higher nutrients in the organically grown.*

Comparisons of analyses of archived samples from **conventional** and **organic** production systems demonstrated statistically higher levels ($P < 0.05$) of quercetin and kaempferol aglycones in organic tomatoes. Ten-year mean levels of quercetin and kaempferol in organic tomatoes [115.5 and 63.3 mg g(-I) of dry matter (DM)] were **79 and 97% higher** than those in conventional tomatoes (64.6 and 32.06 mg g(-I) of DM), respectively. [Mitchell AE et al. Ten-year comparison of the influence of organic and conventional crop management practices on the content of flavonoids in tomatoes. *J Agric Food Chem.* 2007 Jul 25;55(15):6154-9.]

In a nutshell, the ideal human diet is made up of **pure** (not doctored with salt, citric acid, isolated soy protein, sodium caseinate, monosodium glutamate, BHT, BHA, or any of hundreds of other possible chemicals), **fresh** (not bottled, canned, frozen, packaged, altered, chemicalized, dried, fermented) **whole** (not juiced, fractionated, isolated, dehydrated, powdered, floured) **organic** (not treated with fungicides, herbicides, pesticides, irradiated) **plant foods** (rich in thousands upon thousands of protective compounds Nature put there for you). Eat mostly raw, but you can also sauté, broil and steam your food, chop it and combine it together, add herbs and pepper, use organic extra virgin olive oil or real butter, and even spice it up with a little organic vinegar or lemon juice. But know that every step further than these from the foods remaining in their "God-given-state" is a step in the wrong direction.

12 - No Nuts, Seeds, Chocolates, Glutenous Grains

Tissue culture studies have demonstrated a beneficial effect on **viral replication** when the amino acid ratio of arginine to lysine **favors arginine**. This means that high arginine foods encourage the growth of viruses. A body damaged by mercury means cells that are damaged and vulnerable to where bacterial, fungal and viral infections are commonly seen in chronic diseases. Again, the disease isn't *caused* by the infection, the infection is taking advantage of cells being diseased.

The good news is that a predominance of lysine to arginine suppresses viral replication and inhibits cytopathogenicity of herpes virus. Poultry, beans, eggs, fruits and vegetables have more lysine than arginine. There are other foods like dairy products that are also higher in lysine, as is fish. Unfortunately dairy products produce too much mucous, and provide the perfect breeding ground for infections (I have found without fail that colds and flu are far worse in people who consume dairy regularly) and fish is tainted with mercury almost without exception. Gelatin, chocolate, carob, coconut, oats, wholewheat and white flour, peanuts, *all nuts and seeds*, soybeans, and wheatgerm all have more arginine than lysine. [http://www.herpes.com/Treatment.shtml] Below is just a reminder that we want to do everything in our power to *not* contribute to the growth of viruses.

> ...the study revealed a high frequency of **varicella zoster virus** DNA in the cerebrospinal fluid of patients with **MS**, suggesting a possible role of this virus in the pathogenesis of MS. [*J Med Virol* 2007 Feb;79(2):192-9.]

Another problem with grains is that, as outlined in Chapter 4 *Parasites,* bad bacteria in the gut will feast upon glucose and create endotoxins that are highly inflammatory, even deadly. You will read articles and studies that talk about "whole" grains being healthful. They are *more* healthful than refined grains only with regard to nutrient content. Refined carbohydrates means man has taken away protective fiber, and broken down larger sugar molecules into the simpler glucose molecule. Generally, the more unrefined a carbohydrate is, the better. However, that said, *any* grains are too high in arginine, and even whole and unrefined will break down and ferment if left in the gut long enough to do so. People with mercury damage, chronic inflammatory problems, a damaged intestinal lining (seen in everyone with mercury damage, psoriasis, migraines and MS), chronic pain, and who don't *eliminate* as much as they consume – would do well to avoid grains altogether.

13 - No Free Glutamates

The research is clear – excess glutamates wreck havoc – but *especially* in people whose bodies and brains have been damaged by mercury. So my question is, why are food manufacturers adding free glutamates to our food supply *secretly* by the tons every year? Food manufacturers have over 40 glutamate *sources* so that they can "hide" glutamates in their products. This is because they are not required by the flawed FDA to list MSG as long as it is within another ingredient! Go to www.truthinlabeling.org to get the list.

Studies done on glutamates are most often done on glutamates created within the body. To be sure, this is a problem in people whose glutamatergic system has been damaged by mercury. However, there is an equal, if not greater, concern about the tons of free glutmates being added to nearly every seasoned and processed food.

14 - Daily Sunshine

Get at least 15-20 minutes of bare-skin sun. Bare skin means no makeup or sunblocks.

Although the evidence that **vitamin D3 is a protective environmental factor against MS** is circumstantial, it is compelling. This theory can explain the striking geographic distribution of MS, which is nearly zero in equatorial regions and increases dramatically with latitude in both hemispheres. It can also explain two peculiar geographic anomalies, one in Switzerland with high MS rates at low altitudes and low MS rates at high altitudes, and one in Norway with a high MS prevalence inland and a lower MS prevalence along the coast. [Proceedings of the Society for Experimental Biology and Medicine, Vol 216, 21-27, Copyright © 1997 by Society for Experimental Biology and Medicine]

The most important reason you need daily sunshine is so your body can make Vitamin D. Vitamin D is a "precursor hormone", which means it is the building block of hormones. Vitamin D precurses a powerful steroid hormone in your body called *calcitriol*. Vitamin D promotes normal cell growth and differentiation throughout the body – very important in psoriasis. Vitamin D is a key factor in maintaining hormonal balance and a healthy immune system. Everyone knows that Vitamin D is essential for bones and teeth health, but few know that Vitamin D assists in the buildup and breakdown of healthy tissue.

The very best way to get Vitamin D is from sunshine on bare skin (no sunblock). In as little as a couple of hours per week (preferably done in 15-20 minute per day sessions) your body can synthesize more than 20,000 IU of vitamin D. The reason it is better to get from the sun than in a supplement, is because when you synthesize your own as God intended, your body shuts off synthesis when you have enough. If you were to simply take 20,000 units in a supplement, it could prove toxic if you don't need that much.

You would have had to be living under a rock in 2007-2008 to not have heard that Vitamin D actually protects *against* cancers like breast cancer, prostate cancer and colorectal cancer. With regard to skin cancer, it is not sun itself that causes skin cancer, but weak cells that are unprotected by antioxidants, and also mutations in cells that allow them to proliferate unchecked (such as the mutations caused by cadmium from cigarettes, mercury or other toxic metals). In fact, epidemiological studies show that even in cultures where sun exposure is limited, skin cancers have more than doubled in less than 10 years! The truth is, as with other areas of health, we must completely eliminate toxic exposure, such as to mercury, and we must supply the body with copious amounts of nutrients internally, that God in His wisdom has put in pure, fresh, whole, organic plant foods.

Much study has been done on the herb *Polypodium leucotomos* fern sometimes called "Fernblock". Scientists have found that 500-750 mg. per day has been shown to protect human skin from sunburn, and thus cell death. The active components – you guessed it – are phytochemicals! Check out the study in the box below, as you may recognize some of those "phenolic compounds" from the phytochemicals list provided in this chapter. For example chlorogenic acid is obtained by eating pineapples. Again we see where God in His wisdom has given us everything we need in pure, fresh, whole, organic plant foods, to nourish and protect us. In addition, "Fernblock" protects cells against DNA damage, as well as oxidant activity from both natural and ultraviolet light. Anyone who has ignored God's laws for years would do well to take this supplement, especially if they've had problems with sun damage, and especially skin cancer. "Fernblock" is available at www.lifeextension.com or by calling 1-800-544-4440.

Fernblock, an aqueous extract of the aerial parts of the fern *Polypodium leucotomos* is used as raw material for topical and oral **photoprotective** formulations. **Phenolic compounds** were identified as 3,4-dihydroxybenzoic acid, 4-hydroxybenzoic acid, vanillic acid, caffeic acid, 4-hydroxycinnamic acid, 4-hydroxycinnamoyl-quinic acid, ferulic acid, and five chlorogenic acid isomers. [*Methods Find Exp Clin Pharmacol.* 2006 Apr;28(3):157-60. Industrial Farmaceutica Cantabria, Arequipa I, Madrid, Spain]

---

15 - Keep Activated Charcoal On Hand At All Times

My husband and I were poisoned by **solanine** from green potatoes – yet it was quickly and completely turned around by activated
charcoal. Charcoal adsorbs thousands of pollutants as well as different microbes. "Adsorb" means the charcoal particles take the other
molecule to itself – is "attracted to it". "Absorb" means it consumes
it and the "two become one" after a fashion. Charcoal's function is
one of "adsorbtion", and it has an almost singular affinity for nearly
every poison known to man. This means that it actually attracts atoms
or molecules to its own molecules' surface. Then the toxic substance
can be carried out of the body without harming the one who was
poisoned.

God gave us charcoal and we'd be very wise, indeed, to make continued and complete use of it. What exactly is charcoal? Charcoal is
the ashes from vegetable or animal source (bone ashes are considered
to be the best of all). Of course charcoal ashes are created from burning the substance (wood or bone).

If a child swallows a bottle of aspirin or some other poison, and
you rush him/her to the hospital, the hospital will mix a "slurry" of
charcoal in a soda like drink and feed it to your child. Did you know
that? But this has to be done within an hour of the child ingesting the
poison (the sooner the better). So why don't you do it yourself within
minutes? There is no good reason *not* to. Charcoal is available, cheap
and completely non-toxic. You cannot give anyone too much.

Charcoal is effective against nearly every poison as well as infection. In
the "Recommended Reading" section I suggest that you get *Charcoal Rem-
edies.com: The Complete Handbook Of Medicinal Charcoal and Its Applications*, by
John Dinsley. This book should be your "Bible" on Charcoal use. Speaking
of the Bible – God said:

> Then someone who is ceremonially clean will gather up the **ashes** of the
> heifer and place them in a purified place outside the camp. They will be
> kept there for the people of Israel to use in the water for the purification
> ceremony…This is a **permanent law** for the people of Israel…Numbers
> 19:9

...**salmonella** was effectively adsorbed by the **activated charcoal**. [Watarai S et al. Eliminating the carriage of Salmonella enterica serovar Enteritidis in domestic fowls by feeding activated charcoal from bark containing wood vinegar liquid (Nekka-Rich). *Poult Sci* 2005 Apr;84(4):515-21.]

...**activated charcoal dressing** containing **silver** control infection and reduce healing times (of **wounds**), eliminating bacterial barriers. [Verdu Soriano et al. Effects of an activated charcoal silver dressing on chronic wounds with no clinical signs of infection. *J Wound Care* 2004 Nov;13(10):419, 421-3.]

A long-standing method of controlling toxins of many types is the use of high surface area adsorbents, such as **activated charcoal**. Recent data suggest that activated charcoal may offer specific advantages in **topical wound management** through its effects on bacterial toxins. [Ovington L. Bacterial toxins and wound healing. *Ostomy Wound Manage.* 2003 Jul;49(7A Suppl):8-12]

34 children with gastrointestinal diseases of infectious, allergic and mixed etiology were examined.....probiotic preparation Bifidumbacterin forte containing **live bifidobacteria** adsorbed on **activated charcoal** into the complex therapy of digestive tract diseases ensured a **decrease in the detection rate of endotoxinemia** [Lykova EA et al. Bacterial endotoxinemia in children with intestinal dysbacteriosis *Zh Mikrobiol Epidemiol Immunobiol.* 1999 May-Jun;(3):67-70.]

In a TBN movie about the prolific hymn lyricist Fanny Crosby (born 1820) there was a cholera epidemic. I couldn't help but think how if everyone had only been bathed in and drank solutions of charcoal very few would have died. As it was, hundreds died. Cholera is a bacterial infection that gets into the intestines and causes bloody, even deadly diarrhea with extreme dehydration. It is common in countries with dirty water supplies.

> We have seen how quickly and effectively charcoal can work in the much more difficult later stages of **cholera**, even when far from a clinic. We have listened to stories of severe **dysentery** and food poisoning **responding quickly to charcoal** when taken orally and when applied as a poultice. We now have sufficient information to expect charcoal to work just as well for us and for our children in similar emergencies. [John Dinsley, Charcoal Remedies.com pg 166]

John Dinsley has travelled the world, and is an expert on charcoal. He says "we now have sufficient information to expect charcoal to work just as well for us" because in parts of the world that don't have access to "modern" medical care, they are using the miraculous and inexpensive charcoal *first* and saving lives every day with it. America has all but forgotten it. Everyone needs to keep activated charcoal in their homes. If your child or grandchild swallows a bottle of baby aspirin *give them charcoal immediately.* If you wait until you get to the hospital, it could be too late.

Indeed, when you have any kind of infection, or believe you've ingested any kind of poison – turn *first* to charcoal – God's purifier. From a few capsules to a drink made with tablespoons of the powder, you can't get too much. Typical dose to counteract a poisoning would be about two tablespoons mixed in a liquid. In Dinsley's book (see list of recommended reading, Chapter I) he lists both the many ways to use charcoal as well as the very few times it is *not* the best medicine.

16 - When You Can't Take Something Orally

Many medicines and substances that cannot be handled via the mouth/digestive tract can often be handled nicely as a rectal implant. One problem with oral supplements or medicines is acidity which can irritate an already irritated stomach lining. If you have a sensitive stomach, excessive acid or damage, this method may be right for you. Another reason for rectal implants is when there is nausea and oral supplements or medications cannot be held down. Obviously you wouldn't routinely take all your supplements in this way, that would not be necessary. Many of your supplements are very healing to the gastrointestinal tract as well. So keep this method within reach for those times when you need it otherwise.

Rectal implants are actually a very common method that dates back to ancient times. Search the internet for "rectal implant" and you will find more information than you will ever need. There are health spas around the world that utilize this as a means for implanting beneficial bacteria (probiotics) as well as wheatgrass and coffee (look up "coffee enema" online). I've done all of these and more safely for many years. Again, you need to know exactly what they are for, and decide if they are something you'd like to try or incorporate into your health regimen. With any medicine or supplement, you simply empty the substance into a little warm water. You draw it up into a 60 cc syringe, insert a foley catheter tube on the end, put KY jelly on the end of the tube, lie down, insert, and push the plunger slowly to insert into the lower part of the colon. Lie and hold the solution as long as you can usually about 20 minutes. *You absorb what you put into the lower part of your colon.* By the way, this is also why not having regular bowel movements contributes to very poor health. When the bowel remains full, the contents decay and produce various bacteria and toxins which are reabsorbed into the bloodstream.

Where to purchase the syringe: www.premier1supplies.com. It is item #553100. But in case you want to purchase elsewhere, it's called: Syringe, 60cc (2 oz) Catheter Tip. They are about $1.50 each. You can wash it thoroughly and use it again and again (same person) until the plunger doesn't plunge easily anymore. Purchase 10 or so at a time. That many should last over a year even with daily use.

Where to purchase the foley catheter that goes on the syringe: www.shopwiki.com You are looking for the Bard Robinson Red Rubber Catheter. It's an "All-Purpose" Urethral Catheter, 22 Fr. The best one has "two staggered eyes" which means two holes on the tip that is inserted into the rectum. They should cost about a dollar apiece and after each use you can rinse with very hot water and the same person can use many times. One catheter, in fact, can last a year or more. You'll know its no longer usable because it will crack on the end that attaches to the syringe, or it will begin to leak. Go online and familiarize yourself with these items in case you decide to avail yourself of this therapy.

Chapter 12
HELPS

Cooked Vs. Raw Foods

Cookbooks are a "dime a dozen". There are cookbooks for using herbs, for eating "macrobiotic", for vegetarian, for low fat cuisine, for diabetics, for various ethnic cuisines and more. What we *don't* need for healing is another *cookbook*. What we need are guidelines of what foods to choose and how to consume them. At the end of this chapter I give you *Four Healing Meals*. This is because *optimal* healing can only occur when you saturate the body with literally millions of molecules of phytochemicals which include unoxidized omega-3 fatty acids, and *cooking* is not part of the equation. Indeed, for healing, we need *raw* fruits and vegetables. When you cook you destroy phytochemicals.

Does this mean you must eat everything raw? Not really. There *will* be times when you cook foods for the warmth, the "comfort", the aromas. But just know that these are *not* ideal foods for optimal healing. The goal of this chapter is to help you:

1) Be able to consume mostly raw, organic plant foods when you want optimal healing
2) Know what you may safely consume, even if not optimal for healing
3) Have your cupboards full of emergency foods (in case of a disaster or the need for something quick) that won't set you back in your healing efforts

One Week Sample Shopping List

If you purchase everything on this list you would have everything you need to make breakfast, lunch, dinner and snacks for two people for one week of mostly pure, fresh, whole, organic plant foods, with only a small amount of other foods (although they, too, need to be organic, and contain no free glutamates). Again, these are added in for convenience or variety.

So on the list you will find some canned foods and juices. Every family should have a cupboard full of "emergency" foods in case there is ever a time you need food storage for survival. But these foods should be without free glutamates and organic as well. In this way, on that one day a week when you come home starving and have to run off somewhere, and you don't have time to stand at the sink washing and chopping vegetables – your "emergency" foods can be tapped into. In fact, you should rotate the emergency foods. As you consume them, replace them with newer products.

In Southern California, these foods are available at Mother's Market, Whole Foods Market, Henry's (Wild Oats) and Trader Joes. Fortunately, even the larger grocery store chains are now stocking a wide variety of organic foods. You will quickly learn what you will be able to obtain where. Whole Foods, however, is usually your best bet for "one stop shopping", if you don't find it a bit more expensive than a well-stocked grocery chain. In Southern California, Vons is a chain that carries many organic foods, but so do some of the other markets.

Important:

If you cannot find the exact same brands where you live, you can go on the internet and get the ingredients to various brand name foods and do a comparison. For example: The organic olive oil mayonaisse by Spectrum Naturals. I Googled: Spectrum Naturals mayonaisse ingredients. Up popped every mayo they have and the ingredients. Below is the olive oil mayo ingredients. As you can see there are no free glutamate sources, and it's all organic!

> **Ingredients** Organic soybean oil, organic extra virgin olive oil, organic egg yolks, filtered water, organic whole eggs, organic white vinegar, sea salt, organic lemon juice concentrate, organic spices.

You cannot simply purchase any of Spectrum Naturals mayonaisse just because you've read the label on one. Another one has soy sauce in it (and thus free glutamates). And then another one has wasabi in it (again, free glutamates). You must *always* read the ingredients on all packaged foods.

SHOPPING LIST

Juices

☐ 3 quart size bottles of organic **juice** (pear, pineapple or apple are best)

☐ 1 quart size bottle of organic **pomegranate, grape or blueberry juice**

Condiments

☐ 1 small container of organic **honey** (try to get the one that is in the "upside down" squeeze bottle for ease of use)

☐ "Real Salt" a natural **salt** with many other minerals

☐ "Nu-Salt" if you have high blood pressure

☐ Organic black **Pepper**

☐ Your favorite organic **dried herbs** (for example, basil, oregano and rosemary)

☐ Spectrum Natural organic **olive oil mayonaisse** (caution: many other brands have a source of free glutamates)

☐ 1 large bottle of organic, **extra virgin olive oil**

☐ 2 bottles organic **rice vinegar** (preferably from brown rice, and "seasoned" is best – they've cut the acidity a bit with a little sweetener)

Dried Fruits

- ☐ I or more pounds of organic, pitted deglet noor **dates**
- ☐ I-3 small packages of organic dried **figs, apricots** and/or **prunes**
- ☐ I or 2 packages of organic **raisins** (we like the little boxes for pre-measured portions)

Cereals, Beans & Rice Milk

- ☐ organic **puffed rice, corn or millet**
- ☐ organic flakes or other of rice, corn or millet
- ☐ 3 half gallon size organic unsweetened (its normal for it to be unsweetened) **rice milk**
- ☐ I bag of organic **brown basmati rice** (and/or any rice of your choice just so long as its organic — *note on rice: rinse well before cooking!*)
- ☐ I bag of organic **lentils** (green/brown) *rinse well before cooking*
- ☐ I bag of organic **split green peas** *rinse well before cooking*
- ☐ 2 boxes organic, no oil, no salt microwave **popping corn** (or organic popping corn for a hot air popper)

Canned Foods

- ☐ Health Valley organic **black bean soup** (Health Valley is the *only* brand I've found that clearly does not have any added free glutamates — *but* this is only true in their "regular" soup...*not* the low salt or low fat line)
- ☐ Health Valley organic **vegetable soup**
- ☐ Health Valley organic **lentil soup**
- ☐ 4 cans of organic **garbanzo beans**
- ☐ 4 cans of organic **kidney beans**
- ☐ Canned, packed in their own juice, organic **pineapple, pears, peaches**

Eggs & Poultry

- ☐ I dozen organic, free range **eggs** (they can be brown or white)
- ☐ 2 sticks of organic raw **butter** *optional*
- ☐ I tray (containing I-2 pieces per person for 2-3 meals) of natural, no antibiotics, no hormones **chicken [or turkey] thighs, breasts or legs**

Frozen

- ☐ 4-5 bags (usually 12-16 oz.) organic **frozen blueberries**
- ☐ other bags of organic frozen fruits you like, **strawberries, raspberries, peaches** *optional*
- ☐ 2 bags of organic **frozen peas**
- ☐ 2 bags organic frozen **mixed vegetables** of your choice
- ☐ 1 bag of organic frozen **sweet corn**

Fresh Vegetables

- ☐ 7 heads of organic or "no pesticides" **lettuce** (one of the best is the "living" lettuce, like the Boston butterleaf lettuce packaged with its roots still attached, this lettuce lasts for up to *two weeks* as fresh as when you bought it! My family uses a variety of lettuce, from organic romaine lettuce already washed and cut up in bags available at Trader Joes and other markets to whole heads of fresh organic lettuce we purchase at Mother's or an organic farm or co-op nearby.)
- ☐ 1 large container of organic, triply-washed **spinach** use as lettuce for salads and cook in soups
- ☐ 2 bunches or bags of organic **carrots** (we also like the baby carrots already peeled)
- ☐ 1 large or 2 small organic **purple onions**
- ☐ 2-3 organic **yellow onions** (we like the "sweet" ones)
- ☐ 7 small organic **tomatoes** or 1 box of organic baby "grape" tomatoes (this is the first fresh vegetable to go bad, so you may want to purchase only enough to have for the first half of the week)
- ☐ 14 organic **potatoes** or **yams** (or equally divided mixture of both)
- ☐ 7 of your favorite **fresh cooking vegetables** (these can be purchased as they come right out of the garden, or the stores mentioned above sell these already washed and cut up for you!) All organic:
- ☐ **Broccoli**
- ☐ **Brussels sprouts**
- ☐ **Cauliflower**
- ☐ **Green beans**

☐ Swiss chard
☐ Mushrooms
☐ Red or green bell peppers
☐ Zucchini
☐ Cabbage
☐ In season: organic **artichokes**, organic **corn on the cob**

Fresh Fruits

☐ 7-12 organic **bananas** (buy in 2 or 3 in a bunch in varying stages of ripeness if at all possible – but no worries, any that ripen before they can be eaten are peeled and frozen for smoothies)
☐ 14 or more of your favorite fresh organic **fruits** (what is in season) Caution: watch for the word "organic" – many fruits on displays are mixed in with the organic fruits and are labeled "Farm Fresh" or similar.
☐ **Oranges**
☐ **Peaches**
☐ **Plums**
☐ **Papayas**
☐ **Apricots**
☐ **Berries**
☐ **Kiwi**
☐ **Honeydew**
☐ **Cantaloup**
☐ **Watermelon**
☐ **Apples**
☐ **Avocado** for salads

IF YOU'RE GOING TO "CHEAT"

After getting into the swing of eating properly, you'll likely not find much need to "cheat". Mostly, this is because it just doesn't work – *really* cheating and eating something totally off the charts will usually result in more pain or other symptoms. In fact, for optimum healing and health, you'll find that the closer you stick to 100% pure, fresh, whole, organic plant foods with perhaps small portions of organic egg or poultry, the more you will heal, and the better you will feel. But if you find you need to cheat (I'm talking that one snack a week or month - *not* daily) at least make it an intelligent cheat. Below is a list of intelligent "cheater" snacks and foods for people who find they need to "cheat". They are not *ideal* for people working to overcome pain in a brain and body that has been damaged by mercury.

DON'T EAT THIS!	WHY	EAT THIS INSTEAD
"Non-Fat Frozen Yogurt"	Every non-fat frozen yogurt has objectionable ingredients from free glutamate sources in the worst ones, to carrageenan in all of them (highly destructive to your GI tract – promotes Candida overgrowth and "leaky gut")	Breyer's Natural icecream (read the ingredients and choose the ones with the fewest ingredients) or make homemade icecream with all organic, natural ingredients. Do *not* eat the ones with chocolate or nuts.
Flavored Chips, Crackers, and Snacks like "Goldfish"	*All* are riddled with free glutamates hidden in names like "torula yeast" or "natural seasonings". But you will even find pure monosodium glutamate on the label.	Organic chips that contain only organic corn or potatoes, the oil and salt. Nothing else.
Commercial Popcorn	All the "Orville Redenbacher", commercial and "movie" popcorns are full of bad fats as well as being extraordinarily high in salt. After eating the good kind of popcorn you will find that the "bad" kind leaves a waxy substance stuck to the roof of your mouth. There has been some question as to the safety of their popping bags as well.	Purchase organic popcorn and put ½ cup in a plain brown paper bag. Fold the top down several times and place in the microwave for 2½ minutes on high. You may have to experiment as every microwave is different. You can also use those hot air poppers or a campfire popper over the stove flame (my personal favorite). You can purchase an oil "sprayer" and put organic olive oil into it and spray this lightly over the popcorn and season with "Real Salt". Wonderful!

Sodas like Coca-Cola, Moutain Dew, etc.	Each can of regular soda contains approximately 12 teaspoons of white sugar! Most contain phosphoric acid – great if you need to etch paint off of a cement floor – terrible for your body's internal health.	Carbonated juices like "Orangina" or Crystal Geyser Juice Squeeze, or any that are only juice and carbonation. Look especially for organic ones.
Chocolate	Very high in arginine which is the direct precursor to nitric oxide. This is why some people get "headaches" from chocolate as well.	Organic carob or organic milk white chocolate from the health-food store. These are still candy, so reserve for Easter and Christmas and such. Don't buy any with nuts, but you could have the ones that have raisins or rice crisps.
Soy Products	All processed soy generates very high levels of free glutamates. If you are a migraineur you will likely find that eating any kind of processed soy is the sure path to a migraine. For everyone else, the glutamates contribute to your brain and body damage.	Although higher in arginine than lysine, if you consume soybeans, you can only have whole, cooked soybeans. It is in the hydrolyzation, isolation, fermentation and other processing of soy that generates the free glutamates.
Milk	Commercial milk is tainted with pesticides plus hormone and antibiotic residues. Milk was intended for the baby of the animal that produced it. Consumption of cow's milk produces phlegm and produces the ideal environment throughout the body for bacteria and fungus to grow. All heavy dairy consumers will find they have to go through about a year de-phlegming period when giving up milk and its products – but will likely find they have eliminated sinus problems, colds and any chance of pneumonia forever.	Organic, unsweetened rice milk.

Margarine	Margarine is a concoction of altered and oxidized fats. Even if the product claims "no trans fats" (man-made fats that not only do no good, but do direct harm to your body)	Use organic, extra virgin olive oil in and on everything that needs some fat. If you absolutely need or want some butter, use organic (preferably raw) butter sparingly (it's bascially just saturated fat and cholesterol – your body can handle these, though).
Restaurant Food	If someone else seasoned it, they have *most likely* used an ingredient or seasoning that contains free glutamates. You must not consume canned or restaurant soups, salad dressings, pastas, rice dishes, etc. Meats are marinated in sauces that contain free glutamates. Even if you ask them if there is "MSG" *they don't know.* Some will be careless and insist their food does not contain MSG, and you will be the one to suffer when, indeed, it does (in the form of fermented soy, sodium caseinate, yeast products and many more.) Of course that's only one problem with restaurant food – It also isn't organic. Restaurant food is also laden with oxidized fats.	You may eat at salad bars like "Sizzler" or "Souplantation" where you concoct your own plate with only fresh ingredients then use plain oil and vinegar as the dressing. Do not use any of the already dressed choices like potato salad, coleslaw, pre-dressed green salads, etc. For a satisfying meal use lots of beans (like garbanzo) and ask for a plain baked potato (use only real butter or nothing). Don't eat the skin of the potato (pesticides).

| Commercial Cereals like Chex or Cheerios or Total | Read that list of ingredients! You will likely find that the commercial cereal is extraordinarily high in sugar (they hide this by putting half a dozen different sugars, so that none have to be higher on the list than the grain – meaning its more sugar than anything). You will nearly always find a source of free glutamates as well, common is modified corn starch, sodium caseinate or some other "modified" starch. | You are supposed to stay away from grains. Your starches should be potatoes, yams, corn and rice or millet – all low/no gluten, and lower in arginine than grains like wheat. When these are whole, as in corn-on-the-cob, you may include them freely in meals. When they've been puffed or flaked like in cereals, they are now a "snack" for occasional consumption (use rice milk). Sweeten your cereal with a bit of that honey on your shopping list, or better still, an organic banana and/or organic raisins. |

I can in no way be all-inclusive here. If you encounter any temptation to stray from the ideal diet for optimum healing, you now know the "rules". Above all, *never* should you consume anything with free glutamates; and *never* should you submit yourself knowingly to any mercury ingestion (such as that in fish or other sea products).

FOUR HEALING MEAL CHOICES

Each of the four meal choices below represent a meal that is compatible with *optimum* health and healing. When my husband and I are at home, we choose from one of these four meals.

As I said previously, cookbooks are readily available, and you can even get free recipes on the internet. What you need to concentrate on for genuine healing are raw, organic plant foods. When you eat three meals daily of mostly to all raw, organic plant foods, and only use the alternative meal as described below, you will be supplying your body with all the healing phytochemicals it needs, and none of the excess sugars, uric acid, pesticides, glutamates, acid ash, phytates, high argin-ine, etc., that interfere with healing.

FLAVONOID-RICH SMOOTHIE

1½ cups organic juice (I prefer pineapple or pear)
4-5 ice cubes
1 cup organic frozen blueberries
1 whole, ripe organic banana, peeled of course
1 teaspoon organic honey

Put all ingredients into the blender and blend until smooth. Have a "sunny-side" up egg with this to get protein. We also keep hard-boiled eggs on hand for protein when freshly-cooked ones aren't pos-sible. We generally have this as a mid-day snack, though, not a meal – thus no egg needed.
Makes two 12 ounce smoothies

PHYTONUTRIENT SALAD MEAL

1 organic carrot, shredded or chopped fine
1 small chunk organic purple onion, chopped fine
1 organic tomato, cut up in bite-size chunks
1 cup organic frozen peas, thawed (or ½ cup fresh organic peas out of the pod)
½ can organic garbanzo beans
1 head of favorite organic leafy lettuce (not head lettuce) like Boston, Spinach or Romaine washed and cut or torn up into bite-size pieces
Organic, extra virgin olive oil, and organic rice vinegar
Organic garlic powder or fresh garlic and "Real Salt"
Optional: ¼-½ organic avocado per person

Divide ingredients evenly into two quart-size bowls. Toss with 2 mea-suring tablespoons organic extra virgin olive oil and 2 measuring table-spoons of organic seasoned rice vinegar. Now season with your garlic powder or salt "to taste". If you like, fresh organic garlic can be used instead of the powder form — squeeze half a clove on each salad. This is our main meal every day.

Makes two quart-bowl size salads

ORGANOSULFIDE, INDOLE-RICH COLE SLAW

½ head organic cabbage, shredded fine
2 organic carrots, peeled, shredded fine
¼ large organic red pepper, minced
⅛ chunk of an organic purple onion, minced
1 stalk organic broccoli, flowerettes only, chopped into tiny pieces (yields about ½-¾ cup of small broccoli pieces)

Dressing: 2 tablespoons organic mayonaisse (like Spectrum Naturals with olive oil), 4 tablespoons organic rice vinegar, 1 teaspoon honey, ⅛ teaspoon organic garlic powder, ¹⁄₁₆ teaspoon organic black ground pepper. Mix well in a cup and pour over vegetables and mix well.

This becomes a complete meal, especially when you add a large yam with organic raw butter.

Makes two pint bowl size salads

ALTERNATIVE MEALS

As an alternative (usually just for variety), but a meal that does not interfere with healing, we will simply gently cook vegetables (our favorites are the "cruciferous" ones like brussels sprouts and cauliflower). We will have this with organic rice or gently cooked organic (free range) eggs (yolk runny) or a piece of chicken produced without antibiotics or hormones. We drizzle olive oil over everything for added flavor and moistness. Then we season with a little organic garlic, onions and various herbs — a favorite is basil. The options are numerous, and everyone's taste is different. I like my vegetables quite soft, and my husband swears he loves them al dente.

I also fill a glass or stainless steel pot (do not use anything with Teflon or aluminum because they give off toxic metals into your food) half full of water and gently cook chopped onions, split green beans, carrots, cubes of potato, cabbage and cauliflower to make a split pea soup that is one of our favorite alternative meals as well. For variety you can substitute any of these soup ingredients. Simply substituting lentils for the split peas makes an entirely different soup. Season with garlic powder, "real salt", pepper and basil.

Eat at *least* three raw meals to every one that is cooked. For snacks eat fresh, raw, organic fruits.

TESTING FOR HEAVY METALS

You will need to educate yourself *and* your doctor that you cannot test accurately for mercury, lead, cadmium, etc., using a routine blood or urine test. Get information by "Googling": **DMSA challenge test for heavy metal poisoning.** This test has been done safely and effectively for decades. It involves taking 300 mg to 1,000 mg (according to your body weight) of **DMSA** and collecting urine before and after the drug. DMSA pulls heavy metals out of tissues to be dumped into the urine. This is the only way an accurate assessment can be made. These tests are done at www.greatplainslaboratory.com *and* www.doctorsdata.com (urine toxic metals test). You will need your doctor to obtain the kit and prescribe the test.

JUST FOR FUN QUIZ!

Readers of this book have made such comments as, it was "heavy reading", or "deep", and they wondered if they "got it all". Therefore, I've included a little "Quiz" with the intention of showing you that you *did* "get it". That is, you learned the important information needed to help prevent and deal with neurological and painful diseases. After reading this book, you most certainly should be able to answer the following questions. These questions are in the same order in which they are found in the book, chapters one through nine.

Answers Found In The Introduction:

1. Who are the only people who will likely fully comprehend the truth taken from science, statistics, and experience, as set forth in this book? a) elderly people b) people with cancer c) young people with pimples d) one in every two people e) all of the above one day

2. What does "radical" mean? a) wild and crazy b) arising from or going to a root or source c) contrary to what is acceptable

Answers Found In Chapter 1

3. What was the author's "variable" that led to her illnesses? a) genes b) bad diet c) mercury

4. What do most health and medical books say is the cause of your illness? (summed up in 3 words) a) lack of exercise b) too much stress c) need for water d) of unknown etiology

5. What is the "thorn" in psoraisis, migraines and multiple sclerosis? a) a splinter b) lack of medical care c) need for a miracle drug d) mercury

6. We have recently (2007-2008) found an alarming number of imports from China, tainted with what? a) PCB b) arsenic c) vitamin C d) lead

7. Where does healing come from? a) good medicine b) surgery c) physical therapy d) the body's own mechanisms such as stem cells and nutrients

Answers Found In Chapter 2

8. The current population of the United States of America as of 2006 is 300,150,750 (300 million). How many of these people have a devastating disease? a) 10 million b) one in 100 c) 295,000 d) at least one in every two

9. What is causing our current "healthcare crises"? a) because people don't have medical insurance b) because healthcare

costs are too high c) because mercury, glutamates and pesticides (and more) are causing every other person to be chronically ill

10. What is our most prevalent and deadly pollutant? a) arsenic b) lead c) plutonium d) mercury

11. Glutathione is a very important detoxifier in the body. Why is supplementing pure glutathione most likely not a good idea for people with damaged brains? a) it works too well b) you can't buy it in a supplement c) it costs too much d) it breaks down releasing free glutamine which supplies free glutamate

Answers Found In Chapter 3

12. List the Center For Disease Control's three most toxic substances people can encounter any given day a) plutonium, uranium and radon b) arsenic, lead and mercury c) pesticides, melamine and PCBs

13. What substance that caused the death of four infants and injury to 50,000 others is being found in many foods from China (latest article October, 2008)? a) lead b) mercury c) MSG d) melamine

14. What is one highly toxic metal added to gold crowns? a) mercury b) aluminum c) nickel

15. What is the name of the "chemical plasticizer" that disrupts the body's hormones, and has been shown to create a hormonal situation in the body where males don't feel male (among other things)? a) androgen b) estrogen c) phthalates

16. Speaking of "plasticizers", Fill in the blank: "scientists have detected 93% of _____ in humans causing neural and behavioral effects at the current exposure levels." a) MSG b) mercury c) BPA

17. Fill in the blank: Glutathione is perhaps the body's most important and powerful _____. a) protein b) detoxifier c) vitamin d) mineral

Answers Found In Chapter 4

18. Fill in the blank: "at last count there are over _____ antioxidant compounds within phytochemicals category of "phenols" alone." a) 100 b) 1,000 c) 2,000 d) 6,000

19. How is it that we have an epidemic of diseases occuring today? Fill in the blanks: _____ damage your cells; _____ opportunistically invade your cells, take up residence, do great damage; _____ _____ make healing even more difficult if not impossible.

20. Fill in the blank: "_____ is a condition wherein the yeast grow into forms that puncture your intestines causing "leaky gut" a) overgrowth b) infection c) dysbiosis

21. What does Nature create (through thunderstorms and in snow), is found in the air, and it destroys parasites and pollutants? a) oxygen b) nitrogen c) ozone d) moisture

22. Fill in the blank: "Your gut produces _____, when you *feed* grains and sugars to the bad bacteria and fungus residing in your gut." a) vitamins b) nutrients c) alcohol

23. Fill in the blank: "_____ is the end result and insult to your cells and thus, both causes and accompanies disease." a) necrosis b) inflammation c) vasoconstriction

Answers Found In Chapter 5

24. Fill in the blank: "Your doctor (and even you) are so busy gathering up all the "_____" in your disease you never find the "_____". a) information/cure b) data/right drug c) things going on/true underlying cause

Answers Found In Chapter 6

25. Fill in the blank: "_____ (are) the worst dental contributors to disease bodywide." a) dentures b) plaque areas c) teeth whiteners d) dental infections

26. Fill in the blank: "Over _____ different bacterial strains have been identified at the apex or within the pulp chamber of dead or dying teeth." a) 10 b) 25 c) 150 d) a million

27. Fill in the blank: "infections traveling from the mouth and going throughout the body and settling in some far off area - a name for the phenomenon: _____ _____."
a) far off b) bad infection c) focal infection d) none of these

28. Fill in the blank: "Dr. Thomas Rau, director of a medical clinic in Switzerland will say that he estimates 90% of all infections that he has observed in his patients are caused by bacteria from _____ _____."
a) sneezing and coughing b) unwashed hands c) the environment d) dental infections

29. Fill in the blank: It was "Dr. _____ _____'s 1,174 pages of studies based upon 25 years of work by 60 scientists showing how damaging root canals are to the immune system and health." a) Westin Price b) Hal Huggins c) Frank Jerome

Answers Found In Chapter 7

30. What substance found in frozen, nonfat yogurt and other foods, causes intestinal inflammation and damage? a) glutamates b) salt c) carrageenan d) pesticides

31. Fill in the blank: "...psoriasis is a[n] _____ somewhere along your immune and elimination system..." a) defect b) infection c) need for surgical repair d) lesion

32. Glutathione is: (a) a muscle (b) a vitamin (c) a detoxifying agent in the body

33. What level of mercury is safe according to Dr Lars Friberg, 1920-2006, Former Chief Adviser to the World Health Organization on Mercury safety? a) .01-.10 mcg b) 1.0-10.0 mcg c) any level d) no level

34. Fill in the blank: _____ causes widespread damage to DNA, mitochondria, kidneys, neurons, the immune system as a whole. a) a deficiency of vitamins b) lack of exercise c) dehydration d) mercury

35. Fill in the blank: According to the CDC, _____ along with _____ and _____ are the

three most deadly substances on earth. a) mercury, lead and arsenic b) plutonium, uranium and radon c) salt, sugar and fats d) none of the above

36. Fill in the blank: According to the World Health Organization, _____ micrograms of mercury is released into the body every day simply by chewing pressure on dental mercury fillings. a) 3-17 mcg b) .01-1.0 mcg b) 10-100 mg c) 1-5 grams

37. Name the parasite most closely linked to psoriasis (hint: flourishes in and damages the GI tract). a) herpes virus b) tapeworm c) candida d) none of these

Answers Found In Chapter 8

38. Fill in the blank: "...mercury acts as a _____ _____ since there are few pathways available in the body for its excretion." a) neutral agent b) inert metal c) cumulative poison

39. Fill in the blank: "With regard to migraines, studies show that because of mercury damage, the brain's ability to properly utilize _____ leads to a cascade of events the most harmful of which is the excess production of _____ _____." a) glutamate/nitric oxide b) glucose/blood sugar c) estrogen/male hormone

40. Fill in the blank: In a person with a damaged glutamatergic system - the excess glutamates causes a _____ _____ (and this is what causes a migraine). a) bad day b) stomach ache c) neurological firestorm d) none of these

41. Fill in the blank: When toxic levels of glutamate are released, _____ _____ is ultimately released in response. a) vitamin C b) potassium ions c) blood glucose d) nitric oxide

42. Fill in the blank: "...true 100% healing (from migraines) will likely only happen when you can go to your doctor and get _____ _____ _____ injected right into the damaged part of your brain." a) anti-glutamate medicine

b) nitric oxide squelchers c) glutathione producing drugs d) neural stem cells

43. What is the glutamatergic system? a) the system, using glutamates that "fire" your neurons allowing them to synapse b) the system that stops glutamates from damaging you c) the system that breaks down glutamates after their use to recycle the parts into more glutamate for firing neurons d) all of the above

44. Fill in the blank: "Lesions on brain white matter are caused by _____ _____ which are being put into our processed and packaged foods by metric tons every single year." a) bad medicine b) radiation sources c) free glutamates d) salt and sugar

45. Fill in the blank: "We conclude that _____ _____ can be generated by the anaerobic gut flora in the presence of nitrate or nitrite." a) a migraine b) bad karma c) fungal infection d) nitric oxide e) both a & d ultimately

46. Fill in the blank: "...root canals and rotting teeth can be a continuous source of _____ _____ stimuli that cause your *worst* and frequent migraines." a) embarrasing emotional b) bad breath c) excessive stress d) nitric oxide

47. Fill in the blank: It's the premenstrual _____ of estrogen that leads to an elevation of nitric oxide and a migraine. a) fall b) rise c) leveling

48. Fill in the blank: For migraines, eliminating all _____ _____ from your diet is the very first thing you absolutely *must* do. a) bad fats b) sugar sources c) free glutamates d) nitric oxide

Answers Found In Chapter 9

49. Fill in the blank: "There is absolutely *no question* that the pollutant (the "rabbit") causing multiple sclerosis is/are _____." a) herpes b) myelin c) mercury d) doctors

50. Fill in the blank: Dr. Miguel Hernan states "immunization against _____ was associated with a threefold

increase in the incidence of MS within the three years following vaccination." a) the flu b) MS c) Hepatitis B d) measles

51. Fill in the blank: "High glutamate levels lead to central nervous sytem _____ which cause interference of normal neuron signals." a) receptor sites b) loss of neurons c) lesions

52. Fill in the blank: "Your suffering has been contributed to or even caused by the very _____ and _____ people who are supposed to be <u>helping</u>, not hurting you." a) agricultural/grocery b) government/medical c) family/friends

INDEX

Made in the USA
Lexington, KY
30 January 2010